THE COUPLE'S GUIDE TO INTIMACY

How Sexual Reintegration Therapy
Can Help Your Relationship Heal

Advance Acclaim for "The Couple's Guide to Intimacy"

"Bill and Ginger Bercaw represent something very unique amongst mental health practitioners and authors. They, as a married couple, have specialized in helping people reclaim their sexuality. Few professionals share specialties and even fewer focus on sexual reclamation. The problem of reintegrating sex into a marriage after betrayal and trauma is one of our greatest challenges. In this book, the Bercaws have given us a great gift."

— Patrick Carnes, Ph.D., CAS.

"Drs. Bill and Ginger Bercaw have provided a long needed bridge to hope and passion for couples impacted by sexual addiction. Grounded in solid research and clinical practice from both the sexual addiction and sex therapy fields, this book walks couples through a safe, step-by-step approach to rekindling intimacy and sexual passion for those struggling to know where to go next after establishing sexual sobriety. It is sure to become a beacon of guidance for both therapists and couples alike!"

— Kenneth M. Adams, Ph.D., CSAT, author of *Silently Seduced* and *When He's Married to Mom*.

"Written with clinical elegance and precision, Drs. Bill and Ginger Bercaw offer couples a pathway for healing damaged intimacy. *The Couples Guide to Intimacy* gently and clearly offers a necessary map toward integrated partnership, new connection and erotic joy. Their work is essential for couples healing sexual betrayal, inspirational for couples who desire deeper intimacy, and empowering for clinicians who try to help."

— Kelly McDaniel, LPC, NCC, CSAT, author of *Ready to Heal: Women Facing Love, Sex, and Relationship Addiction*

"The Bercaws have created an inspiring and practical intimacy manual integrating wisdom from addiction recovery, human development, sex therapy, and trauma healing. It is clearly and beautifully conceived and explained. It provides a working road map for healing a relationship after the betrayal and suffering of sex addiction. My clients are overjoyed with the results already."

— Mavis Humes Baird, CSAT-S, Founder of *Recovery Sense*

"Drs. Bill and Ginger Bercaw offer a pioneering step-by-step guide for couples struggling to heal and rekindle their sexuality after the crippling devastation of sexual addiction. This important work will offer hope for couples everywhere!"

— Stefanie Carnes, Ph.D., CSAT-S, author of *Mending a Shattered Heart*

"Finally! This *Couples Guide to Intimacy* and the outlined Sexual Reintegration Therapy are long, long overdue. This model truly bridges the enormous gap between individual recovery from sexual addiction and co-sex addiction and the creation of an emotionally and sexually intimate coupleship. What joy! *The Couples Guide* synthesizes the best of clinical trauma and recovery principles with a specific blueprint for marital sexual healing. It's easy to read, engaging, honoring of the individuals and the coupleship, and immensely practical. *The Couples Guide to Intimacy* is destined to become the seminal work in this area. It's the book my clients have been longing for!"

— Marnie C. Ferree, M.A., LMFT – Executive Director of *Bethesda Workshops*, Nashville, TN, author of *No Stones – Women Redeemed from Sexual Addiction* (InterVarsity Press, 2010).

"The Bercaws have developed a unique and highly effective approach to healing the past and bringing hope and intimacy back into the lives of recovering couples. I have always admired their integrity and passion for this work and the tremendous value they bring to such a complicated and difficult area of clinical focus. I would *absolutely* recommend this book to any couple dealing with the pain of sex addiction who desires to move forward in their relationship recovery."

— Jill Vermeire, MFT, CSAT-S, Clinical Therapist, "Sex Rehab with Dr. Drew"

"Drs. Ginger and Bill Bercaw have created a much needed systematic collection of simple strategies designed to accelerate healing from relationship betrayal. They present a much needed map focused on healing at the deepest level- sexual intimacy. In *The Couple's Guide to Intimacy*, the Bercaws address the tender yet complex issues of healthy sexual reintegration for couples crippled by infidelity as a result of sexual addiction. I highly recommend their work as an excellent tool for therapist and couple alike."

— Ken Wells, M.Div, MA, LPC, CSAT, *Psychological Counseling Services* (Scottsdale, AZ)

"What an incredibly valuable resource for every recovering couple and every recovery counselor. *The Couple's Guide to Intimacy* is the first work of its kind – a bridge between sexual addiction therapy and sexual therapy. The Bercaws have provided a step by step sexual reintegration process to help the recovering couple discover the longing of their hearts – true sexual intimacy and fulfillment with each other."

— Dr. Clifford and Joyce Penner, sexual therapists, educators and authors of *Restoring the Pleasure* and *The Way to Love Your Wife.*

Library of Congress Control Number: 2010912650
ISBN: 978-0-9829710-0-0

FOR INFORMATION CONTACT:
Drs. Bill & Ginger Bercaw
California Center for Healing, Inc.
600 South Lake Avenue, Suite 506
Pasadena, CA 91106
(626) 396-9306

Please visit our website at:
www.cacenterforhealing.com
Online ordering is available for this and other products as well.

Printed in the USA
by CreateSpace®
Cover Graphics created by Joel Guinto, joel@mildlysweet.com

Author's note:
Every story in this book is a compilation of true experiences, and each has been edited for clarity. Names, locations, and other identifying information have been changed to protect confidentiality.

THE COUPLE'S GUIDE TO INTIMACY

*How Sexual Reintegration Therapy
Can Help Your Relationship Heal*

Bill Bercaw, Psy.D., CSAT, CST
Ginger Bercaw, Psy.D., CSAT, CST

Introduction by Patrick Carnes, Ph.D., CAS
Forward by Robert Weiss, LCSW, CSAT-S

Table of Contents

Part II: Working the SRT Program

Forward

No one wants to admit that they might have a sexual problem and as a result many good people suffer with these issues in silence and in shame. No couple wants to experience, discuss or have to deal with the pain of broken vows and relationship betrayal, so many couples either "grin and bear it," look the other way or simply break-up. Yet in today's world of instant access to eager strangers and endless porn it is easier now than ever before to trade away long-held values and vows for short term distractions and intensity based escapes. While nearly anyone can be momentarily distracted by the fantasy based comfort that a hidden sexual liaison or online contact can provide, sex addicts and their spouses experience a much higher level of betrayal, loss and pain than most couples dealing with relationship infidelity, often with little direction toward healing.

As most sexual healing and recovery literature is focused on the immediate crisis of infidelity and betrayal, it is rare to find a book such as this, one written with an eye on the long-term goal of couple's intimate relating and healthy sexuality. In *The Couple's Guide to Intimacy,* Drs. Bill and Ginger Bercaw have given both therapists and couples alike a much needed, easily followed, step-by-step guide toward moving beyond the heartache of betrayal and into engagement, genuine communication and healthy, honest sexual intimacy. This book is the long-awaited answer for couples seeking concrete direction, guidance and honest answers toward emotional intimacy and sexual healing. I would encourage any client to take this book home today and get started on the road to sexual healing - for themselves and for their most cherished partners.

Robert Weiss LCSW, CSAT-S
Sexual Addiction: Author, Speaker, and Psychotherapist
Founder, *Sexual Recovery Institute* (Los Angeles, California)

Introduction

As psychologists specializing in treating sex addiction, our jobs require us to work closely with people whose lives have fallen apart. Addiction to anything has that effect, both on the addict and the addict's family. With *sexual* addiction, the effects are especially profound. When the addiction surfaces, there is a strong sense that things will never be the same again. That is undeniably true. Another truth is that there is a built-in potential for healing that would not otherwise be present were it not for the pain of the addiction. Not all couples choose to rebuild from the ashes, and that is always a very personal decision. This book is for those who do, and then often find themselves wondering, "How can we have a healthy sex life after sex addiction? What should we be doing now?"

We have heard countless pleas for guidance in this area. As one woman asked us in her first session, *"I wasn't thinking so much about our sex life when I decided to stay with him- but now I'm realizing how much damage was done. Was I foolish to think we could rebuild our entire marriage?"* The answer to her question (and the many like it we've heard through the years) rests on two key variables. The first is something that cannot be taught: the willingness of each spouse[1] to do whatever it takes to be in recovery. The second is something we *can* teach: a structured approach to building a new relationship from the ground up. That is the essence of the treatment model we developed for this purpose, ***Sexual Reintegration Therapy (SRT)***. It is designed to *guide your recovering relationship confidently toward emotional and sexual health in ways you have never experienced before.*

You may be one of the many couples who want desperately to heal what's been broken. You want nothing more than to say goodbye to dysfunctional ways of relating with each other and to welcome a new way of being in partnership with each other. You want this partnership to be based in trust and intimacy. You want it to flow freely from your living room to your bedroom. Like anything that starts out as an important vision or goal in life, you probably understand that it will only be realized with effective planning.

Sometimes relationships experience the equivalent of a fender-bender or a scratch on the car door. You might get by with a little touch-up paint or even choose to drive it around as it is. But when sexual addiction touches a relationship, it's the equivalent of a head-on collision: There is no question that the car needs to go to the shop. The reality is that because of the damage done to the fabric of the relationship, *you will need help* repairing it and transforming it. Until now, that help has been difficult to find because so little is available for *couples* in this area.

SRT provides the help you will need. If you have a vision for a better relationship, SRT gives you the plan. For those couples who cannot see clearly how a relationship so deeply wounded can be healed, SRT will offer you that hope.

---

[1] For practical reasons and to be consistent, we use the word "spouse" throughout this book (as opposed to "spouses or partners.")

SRT consists of a progressive series of clearly defined experiences that will help you address the core intimacy issues that need upgrading. The structured approach and progressive nature of SRT allows you to lock in the gains that you make along the way. This program will offer you valuable insights and methods you can actually put to use right away. It can be completed in a matter of months, not years.

We have been successfully using SRT with couples in our private practice for many years. We also have been presenting this model to audiences at seminars and professional conferences around the country. The feedback and interest from these audiences and from our clients has reinforced the value and need for the SRT program.

We have heard loudly and clearly from clients using the program that it works for them. People have been consistently finding their ways back to each other with renewed trust and greater intimacy. One husband wrote us after graduating from the program, *"We can't believe how far we've come in the past few months. I only wish we had known what to do a lot sooner."* A woman who updated us a year after graduating from the SRT program wrote, *"What's amazing to me is that we just keep getting better. SRT taught us how to walk through the pain of our brokenness together. We've come through on the other side with a partnership that just wasn't possible before. We know we can keep growing as long as we focus on the key principles we learned from the SRT program."*

The lack of a structured program to help couples get from where they stand currently to where they would like to be has been a major source of frustration for so many couples. It is also why so many of our professional colleagues, including Dr. Patrick Carnes, have been urging us to publish this book. A man who was nearing the end of the SRT program with his wife summed up his experience this way: *"This program has been more helpful to us than anything else we've tried. We knew what we wanted- we just needed a plan that could get us there."* In the end, this book is more than a guide, it is the plan to get you there. We invite you to allow yourselves to be supported by this program, so that you too will discover the healing you desire and deserve[2].

-Drs. Bill and Ginger Bercaw

---

[2] *You should each have your own copy of this book* so you can write your notes and responses in the many sections that require them. This will also allow you the flexibility to complete these sections on your own time rather than sharing the book and needing to coordinate schedules.

Preface

While Sexual Reintegration Therapy (SRT) grew out of our work with couples healing from sexual addiction, it has broad application to recovering couples across all addictions (and even non-addicted populations). The scope of this book, however, *is* squarely focused on the sexual addiction recovery community. The book is divided into two parts. Part I provides the backdrop, setting the stage for a comprehensive treatment program (SRT) designed specifically to address healing around your intimacy. Part II contains the SRT Program itself and is divided into five phases, each with its own focus and objectives.

The basis of SRT rests on multiple foundations. First are the basic elements of sex therapy as first developed by Masters and Johnson. Not only did they propose the "Four-phase model of sexual response," but also the original principles of sensate focus as a means of addressing sexual dysfunction. In the mid 1970's, Dr. Clifford and Joyce Penner developed specific touching, talking and teaching exercises which evolved out of their practice as sex therapists and the work of Masters and Johnson, Helen Kaplan Singer and other sexual researchers at that time. Their Sexual Retraining/Sexual Therapy Program has continued to develop over the years and was the basis of our training in sexual therapy. We, in turn, have adapted several of the Penners' exercises to serve the purposes of the SRT program. Those adaptations will be noted in the context of this resource.

Our training from Pia Mellody has deepened our understanding of how we all tend to experience ourselves and our relationships through the lens of our pasts. Unresolved childhood trauma invariably leads to dysfunctional responses to our adult lives. Addiction and codependence are two prime examples. Pia's work has been influential in shaping our approach to helping couples establish and maintain healthy relationships as functional adults. Her model of functional boundaries is a key component in enhancing intimacy through SRT.

Finally, SRT is grounded in Dr. Patrick Carnes' pioneering work in the field of sexual addiction. His emphasis on deliberately seeking a healthy sexual lifestyle to replace what was once a self destructive sexual lifestyle has been instrumental to our work. He has provided a powerful voice for integrating positive, proactive sexual attitudes and practices as necessary recovery processes. This spirit of hopefulness and self-empowerment across all stages of sexual recovery is a central theme in SRT.

We are deeply grateful for all of the pioneering work from these brilliant thinkers. They have allowed us to create a new resource that is grounded in well-established practices. [3]

-Drs. Bill and Ginger Bercaw

---

[3] Please see the "Recommended Reading" section at the end of this book for the information on the outstanding publications that are available from all of these pioneers.

Part I:
Setting the Stage for Your Sexual Reintegration Therapy

1

Bridging the Gap: Evolution of Sexual Reintegration Therapy

Allison automatically recoiled from her husband's soft touch. "God, I hope he didn't notice that," she thought as she felt a hot wave of shame and dread wash over her. Working quickly to cover her discomfort, she tried to pretend that she hadn't noticed Robert coming in for a kiss. But Allison knew exactly what he wanted. She knew very well that it had been over five months since she and Robert last had any meaningful physical affection. Although she knew she had good reason to feel mistrusting of her husband, she also felt terribly responsible for being so reluctant to feeling any warmth toward him. "Shouldn't I be able to kiss my husband by now?" she thought to herself. She felt absolutely hopeless at times like these. She was still very uncomfortable moving back toward Robert, but at the same time she feared that the longer she resisted, the more likely it was that he would go back to his acting out behaviors. The only thing she felt sure of was that something had to change.

***

Robert did notice Allison's avoidance. It was exactly what he knew he deserved, given what she found out five months ago. He was still ashamed of how he had been deceiving Allison all those years, but at the same time, he was growing frustrated with her foul moods and resistance to any physical affection. "If too much damage was done, I wish she would just say so. Then we could get on with our lives. Does she want to be with me or not? Do I try to give her a kiss or just leave her alone?" The only thing he knew for certain was that something had to change.

Couples working to heal from active sexual addiction have a more challenging job ahead of them than many individuals working to move beyond alcohol and chemical addiction. In active sex and porn addiction not only does the addict's brain become "hijacked" by the repetitive stimulation and then the secretiveness of acting out, the spouse is also repetitively emotionally traumatized by betrayal, secrecy and lies. Some spouses of alcoholics use the metaphor, "It's like s/he's married to the bottle," to emphasize how damaging the alcoholic's relationship with alcohol has been. The damage done to a relationship by sexual acting out needs no metaphor. Betrayal, lies and broken trust strike at the core of any intimate relationship. The long-term healing of physical and emotional intimacy must address the shared scars created by years of lost trust, broken promises and growing distance before returning to sexual and romantic intimacy.

As sex addiction treatment professionals, we hear the painful stories of sex addicts' and their spouse's struggles day in and day out. Couples who have shown the courage to make it through the initial shock, pain and fear surrounding early recovery can feel more alone than ever in seeking solutions to restore intimacy and healthy sexuality. They often have been told (or they assume) that if they simply *work their recovery programs*, their relationship issues, including their sexual intimacy, will resolve themselves. When that doesn't happen, couples often experience frustrations and despair. In reality, the *only* way intimate sexuality will be reclaimed is if it is addressed *directly*. It also requires a level of focus sufficient to support the process of making significant change. A similar level of focus on intimacy and trust is absolutely necessary to create a healthy and intimate way of relating to each other.

The Challenge
One of the greatest challenges facing couples in recovery is learning how to be emotionally and sexually intimate after the relationship has absorbed a direct hit. Our extensive work with recovering couples finds that an overwhelming majority face this frustrating and significant challenge. If you are reading this, perhaps you can relate to some level of dissatisfaction with your emotional and sexual intimacy. You might not be feeling as free and relaxed or present in sexual experiences as you would like. This can be especially true if there was sexual dysfunction or dissatisfaction before recovery.

Concerns like these do not just melt away as you move into recovery. Previously unbalanced patterns of initiation do not automatically become balanced; dormant sex lives do not suddenly become robust; sexual dysfunction does not cure itself. Recovering couples usually have a history of difficulty relating emotionally with each other, and typically struggle to effectively communicate how they are feeling about many things. A subject as emotional as sex is understandably troublesome.

While plenty of non-addicted couples struggle with sexual dysfunction and dissatisfaction, couples in recovery from sexual addiction often develop uniquely complicated patterns. For example, some recovering addicts move in the opposite direction of their addiction by shutting down sexually. The most extreme form of this reaction is called "Sexual Anorexia," which is a complete avoidance and aversion to sex. Spouses, however, tend to move in one of two directions: Some spouses shut down sexually because sex had become too threatening, given the pain surrounding their partner's acting out behavior. Others become *hypersexual*, as a coping mechanism to manage the fear of losing the addict, if the addict's sexual needs are not satisfied.

Additionally, the addict who has been engaging in Internet pornography or Cybersex faces a major obstacle transitioning from the high intensity of stimulation available online to a less intense sexual experience with one's real partner. Spouses and partners understandably often struggle with profound feelings of sexual inadequacy

7

("How can I compete with THAT?"). The reality is they *can't* compete with the intensity that the addict has experienced online. The addict is asked to accept that s/he needs to relinquish some intensity in order to experience more intimacy. The spouse is asked to accept that s/he *is* in fact *enough* of a sexual partner.

Overall, it might seem as if you and your spouse have been walking on opposite sides of a river, each of you perhaps doing great work in your own recovery and even noting some progress in your coupleship. Yet, you might find yourselves still searching for a *bridge to reconnect with your spouse.* You might have a deep desire to take that next step in your journey where you can feel strong in your individual recovery *AND* feel sexually and emotionally connected with each other. If you are like many recovering couples, you have found this level of connection to be quite elusive.

Not Like the Other Addictions

The elusiveness of this connection has been frustrating to many recovering couples for a simple reason: The source of so much pain is also a necessary and vital component of any healthy committed relationship. We cannot just cut out sex, like alcohol, drugs or gambling. This is another reason why recovery from sexual addiction is often more challenging than recovery from alcohol and chemical addiction.

Another challenge is that even if both spouses are open to creating a new emotional and sexual intimacy, there is less information and guidance to be found in the self-help aisle. This is where Sexual Reintegration Therapy (SRT) comes in. SRT fills the gap between "How do I understand what has happened?" and "How does our relationship *get to the other side?*"

A New Frontier for Treatment

Perhaps you have been enlightened and encouraged by some of the reading you have done or workshops you have attended on healthy sexuality. Nevertheless, to put such concepts into action, *and to have them become integrated* on an individual and couples level is another matter. To do this requires an experience that is much different from passively getting knowledge from a book or hearing a speaker. It requires active participation by *actually doing things differently.*

In addition to being Certified Sex Addiction Therapists, we are also Certified Sex Therapists. The latter area of expertise allows us to help couples to identify the sources of their intimacy challenges and sexual difficulties. Even when there is no addiction present, it is a challenge to make room for spouses' different experiences in the bedroom. And, even when we have very effective treatments for any given sexual dysfunction, the treatment plan must be tailored to address the present circumstances and past histories of the two unique individuals that comprise the coupleship.

When it comes to working with couples recovering from sexual addiction, until now, *we haven't had any specific treatment protocols* for improving intimacy inside and outside the bedroom. It has been like life before antibiotics for recovering couples: We have known about the unhealthy agents responsible for the suffering, and some ways to manage the symptoms, but we have lacked an effective program that couples can "plug in" to really experience the deep healing they desire together.

Bridging the Gap

During our earlier years of providing treatment, we noticed a distinct trend: Sexual dysfunction and dissatisfaction treatments that worked well for non-addicted couples were not as effective for recovering couples. These couples needed something to specifically acknowledge that the sexual part of their relationship and the emotional foundations of their partnership had absorbed a severe blow. Not only did this blow do damage, it often revealed pre-existing weaknesses that had not been seen clearly or understood fully.

We realized that the scaffolding for the bridge we had been using with recovering couples (traditional sex therapy) was not supportive and specific enough. We knew we needed *a more specific bridge* for recovering couples. We set out to create an experiential process to help couples find connection in the bedroom while deepening their intimate emotional relationship. *Sexual Reintegration Therapy* is the culmination of our efforts. Now we *do* have a treatment protocol that you can utilize to find what is often experienced as that "last piece of the puzzle:" Your *healthy sexual and emotional selves in the context of a sexually and emotionally healthy marriage.*

One metaphor we use to describe this process of integrating two healthy sexual and emotional selves is a "Bridge to Intimacy." (Figure 1.) When we talk about intimacy, we're referring to the emotional, sexual and spiritual connection that exists as a wide-ranging potential for any couple. It is a useful exercise to contrast typical ways of thinking, feeling and behaving at different places along the path to this bridge and when crossing over this bridge, as is depicted in the following graphic:

<u>Figure 1:</u>

Bridge to Intimacy

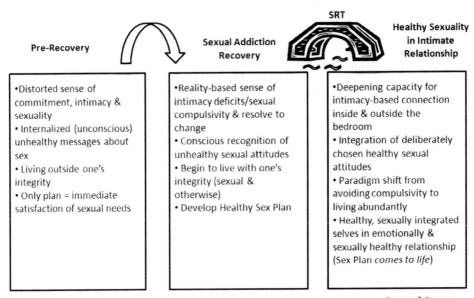

Pre-Recovery	Sexual Addiction Recovery	Healthy Sexuality in Intimate Relationship
•Distorted sense of commitment, intimacy & sexuality • Internalized (unconscious) unhealthy messages about sex • Living outside one's integrity • Only plan = immediate satisfaction of sexual needs	•Reality-based sense of intimacy deficits/sexual compulsivity & resolve to change • Conscious recognition of unhealthy sexual attitudes • Begin to live with one's integrity (sexual & otherwise) • Develop Healthy Sex Plan	•Deepening capacity for intimacy-based connection inside & outside the bedroom • Integration of deliberately chosen healthy sexual attitudes • Paradigm shift from avoiding compulsivity to living abundantly • Healthy, sexually integrated selves in emotionally & sexually healthy relationship (Sex Plan *comes to life*)

Bercaw & Bercaw

9

In Pre-Recovery, typically neither partner has sought treatment; both the addict and co-addict usually have a *distorted* sense of intimacy, commitment and sexuality. Their belief systems around these dimensions are usually impaired due to their trauma histories. Thus, we often see sex-negative schemas (e.g. "sex is disgusting/dirty;" "sex is only good if there is some danger or risk involved;" "sex is my most powerful source of validation" "sex is the most powerful sign of love") as well as core beliefs around feeling worthless, inadequate and unlovable.

Furthermore, while it is the sex addict who most obviously lives outside his/her own integrity, (acting out sexually in ways that result in feelings of guilt, shame and despair), the spouse typically acts outside of his/her own integrity as well. For example, many spouses engage in enabling behaviors, (e.g. protecting the addict from natural consequences of acting out behavior). Other spouses obsess about the addict and develop a lifestyle that revolves around trying to control the addict's behaviors.

In pre-recovery, both addict and spouse (sometimes referred to as a "co-addict") tend to interact with each other through their old wounds. The behaviors they choose to minimize the discomfort they experience in the relationship end up creating more problems than were there in the first place. This cycle repeats itself, and both spouses have their fears reinforced: They are not loveable, not worthy and cannot rely on their partner to meet their needs. One spouse often elevates the other to "My Biggest Problem in the World" status. This has the effect of promoting one's spouse to the role of a "Higher Power." This is the essence of codependence. It is critical that both spouses are able to look through the lens of codependence to see how it is they have been dysfunctional in their relationship (see Chapter 3).

When a couple enters recovery, each can begin to see things more clearly. The intimacy deficits, sexually compulsive behaviors and codependent tendencies are gradually seen from a more reality-based perspective. People have usually made a firm resolution to change their ways, have begun to take responsibility for the pain their behaviors have caused. They likely have enlisted a support system (12-step meetings, sponsor, etc.) to help them with their desired lifestyle changes. They have also started the process of creating better communication. This helps them gain a deeper understanding about how they ended up in so much chaos. To do this, they begin looking at their early experiences, how they learned to see the world, what they learned about relationships and how they came to internalize certain core beliefs about themselves. Many addicts and their spouses begin to develop more compassion for their own past traumatic experiences as well as for their spouse's. (see Chapter 3).

In recovery each person begins to develop more clarity around their personal integrity (both sexually and in general). Part of any thorough relapse prevention involves the development of a "Healthy Sex Plan."[1] This plan is designed to achieve a new perspective around old, sex-negative beliefs and their associated behaviors. A good plan includes not only clear behavioral guidelines around sensuality and sexuality (e.g. "No sexual activities with anyone other than my spouse." "I will ask for a hug instead of waiting to be hugged") but also more life-affirming and relationship-affirming behaviors as well ("I will meditate each morning before I begin my day;" "I will exercise four days per week;" "I will affirm my spouse on a daily basis.") All of these proactive behaviors involve self-care, which necessarily promotes healthy sexuality.

Even people who have received outstanding guidance in developing a healthy sex plan often experience confusion and frustration when attempting to be sexually and emotionally intimate. Many become disillusioned, sometimes re-experiencing the hopelessness they had thought was behind them. The attainment of a deep and meaningful sexual relationship within a safe, emotionally intimate relationship is what many couples desire, but few seem to find.

If you can relate to that desire, you may find hope by knowing that on the other side of the bridge exists a whole new way of life. This way of life is characterized by a noticeably enhanced capacity for connecting with each other. It is on the other side of that bridge that you can experience increasing feelings of hope, safety and competence in rebuilding your sexual relationship. These may be feelings and experiences that you simply have never known before. You can know for perhaps the first time in your entire life what it feels like to embrace a passionate and fully satisfying sex life while retaining your integrity and while being more fully present. You can live a life of abundance, choosing to share yourselves and receive each other as part of that abundance.

When couples are introduced to Sexual Reintegration Therapy, they begin to see a clear path toward approaching what can feel like the final frontier of their healing journeys. Finally equipped with a specific plan to deliberately rebuild and reclaim their sexual and emotional cores, the hope returns, and the journey continues.

2

Who Does SRT Help?

One thing that Mark and Donna had always been able to count on for pleasure was vacation sex. No matter how their bedroom activities might be at home, a hotel room in a faraway place always provided the spark they needed to rekindle their passion. Now, it had been about six months since Mark's bombshell admission about his secret life of massage parlors, prostitutes and Cybersex, and they were becoming more confident in their recovery as a couple. After a mutually agreed upon celibacy period of 90 days ended, they were eager to reignite their passion at one of their favorite seaside resorts. But now this...

Their attempt at intercourse the first night away was a disaster. For the first time ever, no matter what they tried, Mark could not maintain an erection (and Donna could not maintain a positive frame of mind). He felt ashamed and embarrassed, she felt hurt, scared and angry. The second night was no better. Mark decided to ask Donna to do some role playing to heighten the excitement, something they had fun with in the past. But Donna became tearful upon hearing his request: "Why do you need me to be one of your little sex toys now? I'm not enough for you anymore, am I? I never really was enough for you, was I?"

The hope that they brought with them was not around for the return trip home. Instead, they carried home some unwanted baggage: fear, resentment and profound doubt. Few words were spoken on their car ride home, but their internal thoughts were in unwanted sync: "Now what, do we do? Will we *ever* enjoy sex again?"

There are three types of recovering couples that benefit from the SRT program. First are the couples like Mark and Donna having obvious sexual dissatisfaction or dysfunction. They are seeking help from a therapist because their sex life is a state of disrepair. They find it difficult to attain the sexually intimate connection they desire. Typical complaints include low desire, erectile dysfunction, difficulty with orgasm, premature or inhibited ejaculation, intrusive thoughts or images during sex, and unbalanced initiation patterns.

The second type of couple that benefits from SRT may have some sexual complaints, but those are overshadowed by the deficits in their relationship and their emotional intimacy. Typical complaints include feeling undervalued, distant, disrespected, controlled, mistrustful or mistrusted.

The third type of couple that stands to benefit from SRT may not be complaining of sexual dissatisfaction at all. While less common, some couples report that their sex lives are fine. Some even report that they are *more sexually satisfied* after the disclosure or the discovery of sexually addictive behavior. Sometimes this is due to the "honeymoon effect" where one or both spouses crave sexual intimacy in order to feel secure and validated. The sexual validation addresses insecurities around being desirable and loved. This couple may not have the same sense of urgency as the couple with acute or chronic sexual difficulties, but they may value the process of directly addressing their individual and shared sexuality, given its obvious connection to the addictive behavior.

It may be helpful with the third type of couple to use the analogy of a food anorexic: If a food anorexic reported that she really liked food and had favorite foods, it would still be part of her treatment to examine her relationship with food. The goal would be to help her *deliberately decide* how to integrate healthy eating into her daily life. We wouldn't just trust that because she liked some foods, her relationship with food should not be examined. We would not assume that she would figure out how to develop a healthy approach to food. Instead, we would help her develop a deeper understanding of the purpose food serves in her life beyond nourishment, how she has used food as a coping mechanism, and how she developed unhealthy ways of classifying food, such as "good" foods vs. "bad" foods. We would help her develop a structured plan to develop and integrate a new and healthy relationship with food. We would not be comfortable unless this plan was mindful of the emotional component, the *feelings* around eating, as well as the *act* of eating.

This same philosophy applies to recovery from sex addiction. First, we understand that whether or not an addict or partner identifies a sexual barrier or dissatisfaction, that their sexual thoughts, feelings and behaviors *have been affected by the addiction*. Dr. Patrick Carnes has observed, "The addiction has skewed perceptions of sexuality, intimacy, and commitment."[2] For that reason, it is essential that each individual be open to the idea that recovery necessarily involves employing a focused and structured approach. Specifically, couples need to examine how they experienced emotional intimacy and sexuality *before* the disclosure or discovery; how they experience it *now*; and what each person's future *vision* is for things to be different. SRT is the vehicle that allows couples to do this by providing a framework to connect with their sexual, emotional and spiritual selves, and to deliberately decide how to be in relationship with each other through these dimensions of intimacy.

Regardless of what category the recovering couple identifies with, SRT can be an integral part of their shared healing. By the time couples enter secondary recovery, they usually understand that their addiction and co-addiction/codependence reflects underlying *intimacy disorders*. It becomes clear that while the most obvious weakness in their coupleship was the addict's secret life, there is a significant subplot regarding how unhealthy their *shared* relationship was. This is an essential insight shift that any couple who has put together a successful long-term recovery will verify: It is not only a matter of what *the addict was doing,* but of what *we were doing* as a couple that was dysfunctional. However, no matter how dysfunctional the relational dynamics, the addict is always responsible for his/her own behaviors.

Many spouses understandably find it quite difficult to examine their own role in the dysfunctional dynamics of their relationship at a time when they are experiencing tremendous emotional pain. Additionally, many fear that they will somehow be blamed for their spouse's acting out. However, no matter how dysfunctional the relational dynamics, the addict is always responsible for his/her own behaviors.

Focusing on how the spouse has unintentionally contributed to the relational dysfunction would only be advised AFTER the spouse's pain has been validated and honored by the addict. This process takes time and intense work. The outcome is often that spouses feel less "crazy" as their reality is validated, and addicts are likely to develop accurate empathy and healthy shame for their previous acting out.

When a spouse is ready to take the vulnerable step of acknowledging a role in the overall intimacy struggle, s/he takes a much more empowered position as part of the solution. And when *both spouses* are willing to become part of the solution, they can form a mighty alliance against the distance they have been creating in their relationship. SRT is a powerful asset in this alliance to help couples directly address longstanding, distance-maintaining dynamics.

When a couple is able to see more clearly the underlying dysfunctional dynamics and intimacy deficits now exposed via the addiction, the couple has the chance to do much more than just "move on," or "get over it." Rather than waiting for time to dilute the intensity of their pain, they can choose to face their painful realities head on. It is at that time that they can truly begin the difficult, yet rewarding process of building a new relationship grounded in integrity and presence.

Beyond Common Sense

While many couples accept that addressing their sexual and emotional intimacy makes good common sense, it also makes good *clinical* sense. One way of understanding the roots of sex addiction is what Dr. Carnes calls "Courtship Gone Awry."[3] This term refers to the ways that most sex addicts have gone through the stages of courtship out of order, or have taken them too fast. The result is disordered intimacy. Sometimes we see clearly where people have skipped entire stages or have become stuck in certain stages. Stages of courtship include the early stages of "Noticing," "Attraction," and "Flirting," while later stages include "Touching" and "Intercourse." People do not give much thought about which stage of courtship they are in at any given time during a relationship. It's usually in recovery that we learn about such concepts.

Recovery offers two related opportunities for couples. First, you can recognize how your courtship has progressed in a disorderly fashion and the consequences involved. Second, you can take action to develop your courtship in new ways that lead to a deep and lasting connection with each other. SRT represents a way for couples to accomplish both missions. *Recognizing* where things have gone wrong, *reflecting* on how to be in more intimate relationship, and then *taking action* to do so: These are design principles that are foundational to SRT.

14

The SRT program does more than just help you claim and create a healthy and integrated sex life. In order for that goal to be realistic, your emotional foundation must be stronger than ever. *The strength of the SRT program is that it addresses these two tracks- emotional intimacy and sexual intimacy- simultaneously, and thereby facilitates their integration with each other.* It has been described by some participants as a "purification process," where an outdated, dysfunctional system of thinking and relating is left behind, and a new, updated, functional system is installed in its place. You have an opportunity to re-experience your entire courtship, but this time very consciously and deliberately. You are in a position to experience the best version of *yourselves* that you want, in the version of the *relationship* you want.

Figure 2:

Two-Track Approach to Reintegration

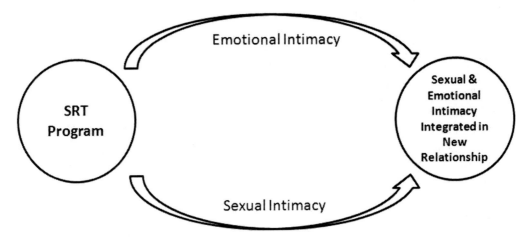

SRT is for

All couples in secondary recovery who are willing to do the required ongoing work of recovery can benefit from SRT. In secondary recovery, both spouses have moved beyond the point of recurrent acting out behaviors and have broken through shame and denial of their painful realities. In other words, you now see more clearly how you had been acting in dysfunctional ways before entering recovery. You have been actively working your recovery programs and noticing positive changes.

The recovering addict has been diligently embracing a new system of proactive behavior while surrounded by support including many of the following activities:
- 12 step meetings (SAA, SA, SLAA, SRA, CR, etc)
- Daily contact with sponsor (and working the 12 Steps with a sponsor)
- Individual Therapy
- Group Therapy

- Reading books on sex addiction, codependence and other identified areas of compulsivity
- Reading books on healthy sexuality
- Making one's therapist and sponsor aware of all past acting out behaviors
- Making a formal *disclosure* to one's spouse/partner of the whole history of acting out behaviors
- Making amends to one's spouse and others hurt by consequences of sexually compulsive behaviors
- Utilizing the latest and most comprehensive recovery resources (e.g. *Recovery Start Kit*; *Recovery Zone*; *Facing the Shadow*; *Ready to Heal*; *Erotic Intelligence*; *No Stones, etc.*)
- Pursuing intensive outpatient or inpatient treatment (if necessary)
- Developing a comprehensive Relapse Prevention Plan with help from therapist and sponsor
- Addressing the physical component of addiction (including completing an Arousal Template Assessment)
- Completing a Courtship Inventory
- Moving toward more active participation in a culture of support (performing program service; participating in fellowship outside of group meetings)
- Developing daily practices such as meditations, exercise and journaling in order to elevate recovery focus

The addict's recovering spouse/partner has also actively pursued his/her own recovery by doing many of the same things including:
- 12 step meetings (COSA, S-Anon, CODA, Al-Anon etc)
- Daily contact with sponsor (and working the 12 Steps of S-Anon/COSA/CODA with a sponsor)
- Individual Therapy
- Group Therapy
- Reading books on sex addiction, codependence to educate and support oneself.
- Reading books on healthy sexuality
- Making amends to spouse and others hurt by consequences of co-addictive and codependent behaviors
- Completing a Courtship Inventory
- Utilizing the latest and most comprehensive recovery resources (e.g. *Mending a Shattered Heart, Shattered Vows, Deceived*)
- Pursuing intensive outpatient or inpatient treatment (if necessary)
- Formulating and presenting a First Step that explains his/her participation in the relationship with the addict (with help from therapist and sponsor)
- Moving toward more active participation in a culture of support (performing program service; participating in fellowship outside of group meetings)
- Developing daily practices such as meditations, exercise and journaling in order to elevate recovery focus

A Word to Spouses and Partners

If you are in a marriage or committed relationship with a sex addict and do NOT identify yourself as a co-addict or codependent you are in a tough spot. While we are not invested in any particular labels, we are *highly invested* in furthering your understanding of how you *chose* an addict as a partner and tolerated much dysfunction over the course of your relationship. It is certainly true that some addicts are quite skilled in keeping their secret life a secret. Yet, no matter how skilled they are, there are characteristics that addicts possess that are not consistent with maintaining healthy, emotionally rich and meaningful relationships- characteristics that you have probably been living with:

- *Addicts struggle with closeness.* They do not let others know much about them beyond a superficial level. They also do not seem to have much interest in knowing others beyond a superficial level. Reasons for this are many, but in a nutshell, they learned long ago that to be open and vulnerable enough to allow for close, intimate relating is quite threatening. In order to cope with this "threat," they have learned to employ avoidance strategies to maintain a comfortable buffer of distance between themselves and others. You likely have felt this distance.

- *Addicts struggle with honesty.* Even on the "small stuff," many addicts have tendencies to play fast and loose with the truth. (e.g. Telling you the supermarket was out of your brand of yogurt when the truth is he forgot to buy it; "Forgetting" to mention the plans to play poker with the guys tonight.) You likely have felt the effects of your spouse's dishonesty, either on small stuff, major issues, or both.

- *Addicts struggle with moderation.* Usually there are domains of the addict's life other than the sexual in which s/he finds it difficult to practice moderation. For some, it involves overworking, overeating, or exercising excessively. Often the excess is masked as passion for a hobby (e.g. spending evenings and weekends fixing computers or playing video games; obsessively pursuing collectible items). Sometimes the excess is apparent in the way the addict approaches finances, either in an over-restrictive or a careless or risk-taking manner. In other cases, the addict has struggles with time, always running late or in the other extreme, being especially rigid about schedules. You have likely felt the effects of your spouse's struggle with living in moderation.

- *Addicts struggle with boundaries.* Addicts typically lack a sense of how to practice respectful boundaries with others. This deficit extends to all areas of the addict's life from how much information to share with others, to how much physical touch is appropriate (e.g. hugs) or what forms of humor or other comments are appropriate relative to the situation. You have likely noticed your spouse's lack of appropriate boundaries in at least one domain of his/her life.

- *Addicts struggle with interdependence*: Interdependence refers to how we get our needs and wants met in relationship and how we decide to be available to help others get their needs and wants met. Most people who struggle with addiction have a difficult time *knowing* what they want, *expressing* what they want, or struggle with both. They also struggle with deciding *how* to be available to others. This makes relating with them challenging because they tend toward two extremes: Either they are "needless and want-less" (e.g. "No, I'm fine with

17

whatever you want to do.") or on the other extreme, needy and demanding ("You haven't said 'I love you' all day, are you mad at me?"). In recovery, many come to understand that their addictive behaviors grew out of the distorted belief that they cannot count on others to meet their needs. It is likely that you have felt frustrated by your spouse's challenges around your needs and wants as well as his/her own needs and wants.

- *Addicts struggle with anger*. Individuals who struggle with addiction often walk around feeling victimized by others. In their minds, they have been treated unfairly, have been taken advantage of, have been done wrong by others, and have been shown disrespect. Sometimes there may be a kernel of truth to their perceptions that others have not behaved fairly or properly. But when their reaction to that perception is to "right the wrong" by using a revenge strategy, relating becomes quite difficult. Revenge strategies range from giving someone the "cold shoulder" or "silent treatment" to raging outbursts of attacking language or even physical violence. The belief behind these behaviors is, "Because you have rejected me or offended me, I have the right to get back at you and punish you, to even the score." This is what Pia Mellody calls "offending from the victim position." It is likely that your spouse has felt victimized by you and has used some revenge strategies to cope with feeling offended or rejected.

As you read these characteristics, did you notice some that may apply to you as well? If so, this would not only be normal, but potentially very helpful in your individual and couples healing. Taking your *own* inventory of dysfunctional tendencies will allow you to join forces with your spouse to create that "mighty alliance" mentioned earlier. It is perhaps best said by Co-Sex Addiction expert and author, Dr. Stefanie Carnes:

> "Isolating those areas of the relationship where you compromised your values or gave too much of yourself will help you understand how co-sex addiction applies to you. By learning about addiction and co-sex addiction, you will gain insight into the common dynamics in addictive relationships and discover tools to prevent yourself from being manipulated again in the future."[4]

Owning the label of "Co-Sex Addict" is of secondary importance compared with the importance of seeing how you may have been losing yourself in your relationship with the addict. Resisting this truth limits the depth of healing that can occur in the relationship and within yourself. Embracing it allows you to set yourself free. The rest of this book represents a targeted plan of action for achieving that freedom you have long wanted and richly deserved.

3

"The Story of Our Lives"

Susan couldn't believe how fast her world was spinning. Bob, her husband of 15 years just confessed to having serial affairs and being addicted to internet porn. How could this happen? Susan had promised herself that she would never end up in a marriage like her parents. Her dad was an alcoholic and cheated on her mom throughout their marriage. Susan's mom looked the other way and tried to make up for her dad's absence due to his drinking and philandering. When Susan met Bob she thought she hit the jackpot. Bob was a straight-A student, athletic and very outgoing. He was so handsome and pursued Susan in a way that felt loving and respectful. Bob never pushed sex on her when they were dating and once they were married they fell into a pattern of once a week sex on her initiation. If anything, Susan had worried that Bob was working too hard at the office. He was only 39 and had just been made a senior partner at his law firm. He worked late most evenings and some weekends. Susan missed Bob, and the kids were starting to notice that he was gone a lot of the time. "How did I get here?" thought Susan. "How did it get this bad?"

System Failures

"How did I get here?" and "How did it get this bad?" are two of the most common questions that spouses and addicts ask themselves in recovery. Research shows that addicts and their spouses or co-addicts each develop from similar origins. A landmark study by Dr. Patrick Carnes demonstrated that both groups come from homes marked by trauma. Trauma comes in many different forms: sometimes it is overt, as in the case of physical or sexual abuse, and sometimes it is covert, as in the case of growing up with an enmeshed, distant, emotionally abusive, manipulative or addicted parent.[5]

Carnes looked at common factors in family systems that are correlated with sex addiction. He found that 77 percent of addicts came from "rigid" family systems, meaning that there are strict rules and significant consequences for not following the rules. A child growing up in this type of home learns that they must adhere to the parent's expectations of behavior in order to be accepted "or else." Of course, this is a

19

highly conditional form of love, as well as an unrealistic standard. The child experiences much shame and doubt about the self when s/he acts "bad" or experiences impulses that are not consistent with the perfect, expected persona. Often, what constitutes "bad" behavior in a rigid family system is actually developmentally age-appropriate behavior that is consistent with the child's vulnerability, immaturity, or spontaneity. These homes also tend to carry a sex-negative message, to be sexually repressed and to have high levels of shame about sexuality.

The narrow window of acceptable behavior imposed by the rigid family system sets children up to feel as if they are continually failing to meet an unreachable expectation. Many of these children grow up feeling fundamentally flawed and worthless compared to other people. Similarly, children often sense that the parent does not love him/her as he/she is, and an incredible pain is felt. This leads the child to be hyper-aware of his/her actions as well as the way that others respond to him/her. The child's natural spontaneity gets overwhelmed and overrun by the child's fear of rejection and punishment.

Commonly, children respond to this type of environment in one of two ways. Some try to attain the parents' approval by acting good and perfect. In this situation, the child continually looks to the parents for their approval and happiness to determine his/her self-worth. Of course, this child often feels like s/he is on an emotional roller coaster and walking on eggshells as they are attempting to control the parent's mood and gain the parent's approval by his/her behavior. In this type of an environment, a false self is created as a way to adapt to the pressures of this type of home. While the false self helps to protect the child from the relentless criticism of the parents' rigid expectations, it also makes it impossible for the child to develop a true sense of who he/she is. Authenticity is sacrificed.

This way of relating with others is naturally carried forward into adulthood. Jim, a recovering sex addict said he had an "aha" moment driving in the car on the way to his parents house for Christmas. "It suddenly occurred to me that I had no idea who I was. What did I like? What were my interests? It was like a light bulb went off and I suddenly realized I had been living my life for my parents' approval." Constantly looking outside the self for approval and self-acceptance is a tremendous burden for any child. As adults, such individuals often find relationships to be emotionally draining and not very satisfying. Jim went on to say, "This was a real turning point for me. I felt such a sense of pain and joy at the same time. All at once I saw how I had been keeping my true self hidden from others and now I had the chance to break free. The only problem was I had no idea how to do it. That is when I sought help for my recovery."

On the other hand, if the child chooses to go in the opposite direction of "good and perfect" by rebelling against the rigid expectations of the parents, the child is often a scapegoat and blamed for all the problems in the dysfunctional family. A scapegoat child becomes, as Pia Mellody says, "very good at being very bad." Sandy recalled growing up with her perfect older sister. "My parents thought the sun and moon revolved around my older sister, Darlene. It didn't matter what she did. They thought she was wonderful. And I guess she was; she was pretty, smart, a cheerleader and had lots of friends. I realized at an early age that I would never get their approval because

20

they adored her so much. I finally stopped trying and began acting out by hanging out with the "bad" crowd and doing drugs. At the time I didn't realize I was doing it to get attention. Now I see it as a real cry for help. I just wanted them to care for me the way they did Darlene." There are various paths that lead children to the same conclusion: that they are fundamentally unlovable, flawed, and unacceptable as they are.

As an adaptation to these conclusions, many children develop a "secret life" where they act out their impulses beneath the radar of their parents. This was the case with Sandy. What began as hanging out with the "wrong crowd" and doing drugs, quickly spiraled into excessively flirtatious behavior in high school and clinging to her boyfriends in college. As Sandy described, "I was never without a boyfriend and it almost immediately became sexual. I needed that interaction to know that they cared about me, that I actually mattered. When I wasn't with my boyfriend, I thought about him all the time, I wondered who he was with and if he still loved me. I couldn't relax until we were having sex. Then, when it was over, the cycle would start all over again. That empty hole that I was carrying around was bottomless. I needed more and more sexual attention to feel better about myself. Twenty years later, I see now that I have a problem. It is amazing that I didn't get an STD with all of the unprotected sex. I know now that I need to start feeling better about myself as I am, not based on who I am sleeping with."

Bob, from the beginning of this chapter, also typifies what it is like to have a secret life. When Bob was nine years old he found his dad's stash of Playboy Magazines and other, more hardcore sex magazines, in the family's garage. Suddenly, Bob understood why his dad spent so much time in the garage and why his mom was so annoyed when Dad seemed to be out there for a while. It was that same garage that Bob was sent to sit in for punishment when he misbehaved. Before too long, Bob started intentionally misbehaving in order to get sent to the garage so he could look at his dad's pornography and masturbate. He also discovered the intoxicating rush of adrenaline that accompanied his many successful "smuggling" missions of sneaking a magazine or two back into his room. He could not control how harshly his parents yelled at him, or how severely they would spank him before sending him off to the garage. But he took great pleasure in creating a secret world they would not discover, and he never looked back.

Patrick Carnes also found that 87% of the sex addicts he studied came from homes categorized as "disengaged," meaning that there is a low level of cohesion and low levels of bonding. Everyone in the disengaged family system is on their own in taking care of their emotional needs. Children that grow up in this type of home often feel a profound sense of loneliness and eventually may become mistrustful of others, particularly of the people who are supposed to love and care for them. This failure to bond leaves a deep and painful void. Susan, from the above example, knew this void well and described it as a "constant aching in my heart."

Children from disengaged family systems learn that they can't count on others to nurture, love them and meet their needs. When the necessary care is not available and the pain becomes intense, these individuals become quite vulnerable to looking for other things to fill the void and numb the pain, such as sex, masturbation, gambling, alcohol, food, porn, serial affairs, over-exercising, over-working, even over-controlling others. These outlets provide only a brief relief from the pain, and carry their own

21

consequences that tend to make life unmanageable. They never actually fill the huge void. However, they are dependable and consistently available. Once a person comes to rely on compulsive behaviors to manage pain, s/he tends to need more just to feel "normal".

The disengaged family system profile sets the stage for dependency issues. There is a very low level of cohesion among the family members, and the children in the family often feel that they are on their own to get their needs met. A lack of interest from the parents is felt by the children, and the children end up feeling empty and unworthy of being cared for. This creates quite a dilemma, because children *are* inherently needy and dependent.

When a parent does not provide a minimum amount of nurturance, a child has a few choices. One option is to become overly dependent and needy, basically begging for care and affection. The other is to develop an anti-dependent stance in which the child chooses to rely on no one else to meet his or her needs. Again, these orientations become deeply integrated into a child's psyche and get carried forward into adulthood and into adult relationships. For example, John, a recovering sex addict, recalls his childhood experience of being on his own. "Growing up, my mom was never around. My parents never married and my dad was not in the picture. My mom would go to work in the morning, go out on a date at night and come home after I went to bed. I learned early on that I couldn't count on her or anyone else to take care of me. I remember at age seven making my own meals and getting myself to school. If I didn't do it, it wouldn't happen."

When children grow up in rigid, and/or disengaged homes, they are predisposed to have difficulty with intimacy and with dependency issues. The reason for this has everything to do with the "Core Beliefs" that these environments breed. The most prominent core beliefs an addict carries around are:

1. I am basically a bad, unworthy person.
2. No one would love me as I am.
3. My needs are never going to be met if I have to depend on others.
4. Sex is my most important need.
5. I am bad because sex is my most important need.[6]

The first three core beliefs tend to develop early in life and the last two develop after a person develops compulsivity around sexual behavior.

Similarly, the co-addict develops certain core beliefs about the self:
1. I am basically a bad, unworthy person.
2. No one would love me as I am.
3. My needs are never going to be met if I have to depend on others.
4. Sex is the most important sign of love.

Similarly, for co-addicts, the first three core beliefs are set into motion early in their lives and are foundational for the way the addict and the co-addict experience

22

themselves and others in relationships. Core belief #4 can become more pronounced as a result of discovering the addict's sexual acting out.

These core beliefs are extremely powerful in shaping how the addict and co-addict experience themselves and their relationships. It is crucial in therapy and recovery that the addict and co-addict identify these beliefs and understand how they were developed in their family of origin, and reinforced in subsequent relationships, including with their current partner.

In addition, it is fundamental to the addict's and co-addict's recovery that these unconscious beliefs are exposed for the lies that they are. Each core belief needs to be consciously changed to reflect a true sense of self-love and affirmation. Through the hard work of early recovery, individuals come to believe that:

1. They are lovable.
2. They are valuable and that all humans are of equal value.
3. They can count on others and have a healthy relationship that is characterized by interdependence.
4. Sex is an important need and having a healthy, respectful sexual relationship with the self and their partner is a valuable part of life.

Psychiatrist Daniel Siegel talks about the importance of people understanding the story of their lives, and refers to it as the "coherent narrative." So much of recovery is looking at the messages we received and the experiences we had growing up and making sense of them. However, it is clear that this knowledge alone is not enough. Healing requires an integrated approach that blends the factual experiences that occurred with the important *emotional* memories of the experience. As Siegel states, "A deeper self-understanding changes who you are. Making sense of your life enables you to understand others more fully and gives you the possibility of choosing your behaviors and opening your mind to a fuller range of experiences."[7] This concept is at the heart of recovery, as addicts and co-addicts gain greater self-understanding and expand their capacities for relating intimately with others.

With the help of a skilled therapist who understands family of origin issues and trauma, both spouses can identify the messages they received growing up that helped to create their core beliefs. Some of these messages are obvious. For example, one woman described growing up with a raging mother who would hit her and tell her she was worthless anytime the girl acted in a way that was outside of her mother's rigid expectations. Other messages are more subtle, such as a father offering to help his adolescent daughter with her homework as a way to engage her so he could talk about his frustrations about his wife's spending. In either way, there is a programming effect on the child. As adults, we need to understand how our original programming affected us as children and how naturally we revert to that programming today, despite it not serving us well.

Dorothy, in recovery from sexual anorexia, desperately wanted to make sense of why she enjoyed sex so much before she was married and then felt "absolutely repulsed and terrified" of sex after being married. The system Dorothy described in her family of origin was very rigid and disengaged. She adapted to her parents by becoming "good and perfect." This included making excellent grades, being very polite, and not being sexual with her boyfriends. "My mom was so afraid that I was going to get pregnant and disgrace our family. I am not sure why she was so worried about it. I did everything she told me to just to get her to leave me alone. She was always on my case. One time in high school, I skipped my period. I didn't think it was a big deal because I was always a little irregular, but my mom flipped out. She started interrogating me about what I had been doing with my boyfriend. She actually asked me if I was a slut! I don't know what happened to me, but I got just as angry at her and told her my sex life was none of her business. Well that really escalated things! The next thing I knew she was hitting me and telling me I shouldn't even have a sex life. I knew then and there that she was absolutely crazy and I couldn't wait to get out of that house."

While in college and afterword, Dorothy had sex with her boyfriends and found it to be very exciting and pleasurable. "There was always a little thrill in knowing that I was doing something that I wasn't supposed to." When Dorothy met her husband, she was extremely attracted to him and they had great sexual chemistry. "We couldn't keep our hands off of each other. I just expected that to continue into our marriage. Instead, it came to a crashing halt on our wedding day. I found myself worrying about being sexual on our wedding night, which was very unusual. In the past, we were both very free and spontaneous, almost swept away in the moment of passion. Suddenly, sex felt like a heavy burden and an expectation that I needed to fulfill for my husband."

What followed the wedding was 10 years of pain, confusion, constant arguing, and a near divorce. Dorothy's husband, Kyle was confused and hurt. Before he and Dorothy married, she was open, spontaneous and always willing to be sexual. What happened after their wedding only further perplexed Kyle because he and Dorothy had such a great relationship otherwise. "We are the best of friends. I love Dorothy more than anything in the world but I don't understand what has happened to us sexually. She is never interested in sex and almost seems to recoil from it when I suggest it. I have just stopped asking. During our last fight about sex I told her that I couldn't go on like this anymore in a sexless marriage. That was when Dorothy agreed to go to counseling."

Once in therapy, Dorothy began piecing together the negative messages she received about sex in her family, as well as how physical affection was expressed between her parents. She recalled her mother seeming uncomfortable with her dad's affection, often pulling away from it. She also recalled her uncle making suggestive comments to her about her developing body in adolescence that made her feel very uncomfortable. Dorothy was able to see the evolution of her sexual self throughout the course of her life, including the ingrained belief that sex was something that men took from you. She was able to see the formation of her core beliefs and how sex had become her most terrifying need. After much hard work, Dorothy was ready to shed the old beliefs and was ready to reclaim her sexuality as her own, not the tainted image of it that was passed onto her from her family.

Through her recovery, Dorothy was able to consciously become the author of her own life instead of unconsciously playing out old roles and relating to her husband from an outdated script. For her, this included creating an entirely different way of thinking about herself, her sexuality and herself in relationship with her husband. She

24

was able to see how she had been depriving herself of care and nurturance. She allowed herself to accept care and love from Kyle, including physical and sexual care. An important self-statement for Dorothy was one in which she affirmed her sexuality and claimed her right to sexual pleasure. She reflected, "This all felt extremely foreign, a little scary, and at the same time amazingly liberating. I knew I needed a new way of thinking about my sexuality, but emotionally it felt like a real push-pull. I could feel part of myself breaking free of the old patterns and ways of thinking about sex, and yet a part of me still felt safer hiding from it."

During the SRT program, Dorothy learned how to keep herself safe while being emotionally and physically intimate with Kyle through her functional boundaries. This allowed her to be vulnerable with him, and to feel safe enough to try out new experiences with her new way of thinking about sex. For example, when they started their sensual caressing experiences, Dorothy sometimes felt anxious. She would tell Kyle when this happened and then take a minute to breathe through her feelings and figure out if there was another way to approach the experience with less anxiety. Kyle helped by clearly expressing that her comfort was important to him and encouraged her to let him know how she was feeling. He was very patient and respectful. Although it was challenging for him to see his wife struggling, he was respectful of her feelings and motivated to help move their relationship in a healthier direction.

These types of interactions are pivotal in Sexual Reintegration Therapy for several reasons. First, it takes a great deal of courage for Dorothy to share her reality with Kyle and it implies new ways of thinking. One is that she is of equal value in the relationship and neither of their needs take priority over the other's. They are truly partners in creating their sexual experiences together based on mutual comfort and pleasure. Second, it implies a sense of trust in Kyle that he genuinely cares about her and her comfort. It also involves trusting that Kyle can tolerate Dorothy's feelings and will not try to manipulate her into doing things his way. This sense of trust in Kyle goes against her long held belief that "my needs will not be met in relationship with others." It speaks to the flexible nature of the sexual relationship. Although there might be some initial expectations going into a physical/sexual time together, Dorothy and Kyle have learned to value the ability to be flexible and adaptable in their relationship.

This open, flexible approach is a design principle running throughout all of the Sexual Reintegration Therapy experiences. The relationships with yourself and with your spouse are at the heart of this type of deep healing and change. Through SRT these relationships are grounded in a deep sense of love and respect. The very nature of SRT is abundant and life-affirming. You can understand the effects of your past, take ownership of today, while hopefully anticipating tomorrow. The future is bright. The spirit is hopeful. Let's continue the journey together by beginning to lay the foundation for the change you desire and deserve. The exercise that follows is the first step along this journey.

Story of My Life
(Bercaw & Bercaw)

Purpose & Goals:

The most important story we ever encounter in our lives is our own. One of the great life skills is to know how we came to be the way we are. With this awareness, we are better able to understand why we have the thoughts, feelings and behaviors we do, in certain specific situations and in general. Many of these thoughts and feelings occur on an unconscious level, as they form our "default modes." One of the goals of recovery is to expose our default modes, to make the unconscious, conscious. When we are able to experience ourselves and others more consciously, we achieve a freedom from automatic ways of thinking, feeling and behaving, learned long ago as adaptive responses to challenging childhood experiences.

This is accomplished in two stages: The first stage involves answering questions about your past. It is designed to help you gain clarity on the pieces of your history that you need to see clearly in order to be able to tell that most important story, the story of your life. The second stage is explained near the end of this exercise.

Instructions:

Respond to the following questions as completely as you can. When you are through, read the finishing instructions.

A. MY FAMILY MEMBERS

1. When I was born, the following people were living in the home:

2. My mother was _____ years old. From what I know, this is how she felt about my arrival:

3. My father was _____ years old. From what I know, this is how he felt about my arrival:

4. When I was around my mother I would feel...

5. When I was around my father I would feel...

6. The best thing about my mother was...

26

7. The best thing about my father was…

8. The worst thing about my mother was…

9. The worst thing about my father was…

10. I would describe my parents' relationship as…

11. Something I learned from my parents' relationship was…

12. When my parents had a conflict, they would usually…

13. When my parents had a conflict, I would usually…

14. I had _____ siblings. This is how I would describe each of them and my relationship with each one:

15. The best part about growing up in my family was …

16. The worst part about growing up in my family was…

B. MY FAMILY ROLES

List examples of how you played one or more of the following roles as a child:

Scapegoat- the one who would get blamed, always in trouble, highly criticized

Lost Child- the one who was overlooked, not attended to, invisible
Hero- the family fixer, problem-solver, over-achiever, good and perfect. [4]

---

[4] For a more detailed description of these roles, we recommend, *The Intimacy Factor* by Pia Mellody.

C. MY FAMILY RULES

Every family has a culture of rules or expectations for dealing with reality. Some families talk openly and respectfully about problems, without blame, while others are programmed for fault-finding. Some other families have a culture of silence, where problems are generally not acknowledged. When a problem does surface, some families will deny or minimize its existence through a number of ways (anger, avoidance, controlling/manipulative behaviors, addictive behaviors, etc.). Write about your family rules and how your family dealt with problems. Provide any examples that come to mind.

D. SEXUALITY

1. The messages I received in my home about sexuality:

2. The information I received in my home about sexuality:

3. The messages I received in school (and/or church) about sexuality:

4. My parents' attitudes toward sexuality:

5. My parents showed affection to each other by:

6. My parents showed affection to me by:

7. When my body started developing sexually, I felt:

8. My family reacted _____ (positively, negatively, not at all) to my developing body.

9. Describe how nudity was handled in your home.

10. Were you ever touched inappropriately by an older adolescent or adult?

11. How did you feel about your sexuality growing up and what was most influential?

12. How would you describe your body image?

13. Describe the body image of your same sex parent as you understand it:

14. What messages did you receive about masturbation (and from whom)?

15. At what age do you remember discovering your genitals?

16. Describe your masturbation history including presently.

17. At what age did you have your first sexual intercourse? Describe the situation and your reaction to the experience.

18. How did you decide to become sexual with another person?

19. How did you feel about yourself after becoming sexually active?

20. How do you currently feel about your sexuality?

21. How would you like your sexual life to be currently, including your sexual self esteem?

E. RELATIONSHIPS

1. What did you learn from your childhood relationships with same gender peers? (Such as, "I was liked and accepted by my same gender peers when I was the class clown.")

2. What did you learn from your childhood relationships with opposite gender peers? (Such as, "I believed that I was not very attractive because boys never asked me out.")

3. What did you learn about relationships from how your parents responded to your friendships? (Such as, "My parents encouraged me to have friends over. I learned that friendships are important.")

F. ADDICTIONS

1. Who were the people in your family (Parents, grandparents, aunts, uncles, siblings) that struggled with addictions (drugs, alcohol, sex, spending, gambling, working, overeating, restrictive eating, and compulsive exercise)?

2. How did the family deal with and act toward the people with the addictions above?

3. How were you affected by these addictions?

G. STORY OF YOUR LIFE: What You Have Been Carrying Around

Based on what you've identified above regarding rules, roles, and other influential childhood experiences, what do you think you have carried forward with you as an adult? For example, some people have a hard time asking for what they need or want. They then come to understand that they have carried the belief forward that their needs and wants were not important. Or consider someone who tends to assume that others' negative feelings must somehow be her fault. She might also be aware of a connection between this adult tendency and a pattern of being a scapegoat or enmeshed as a girl.

Finishing Instructions: Use this reflective process to write the "Story of Your Life" as you understand it today. Be patient with this process. It is important to understand that the Story of Your Life will continue to be fine tuned and revised as you continue in recovery and throughout your lifespan. Think of this as beginning point of writing out your coherent narrative.

4

Criteria for Readiness: "Timing is Everything"

Diane knew they had to do something. After years of living in a sexless marriage with her husband, Greg, and after the pain from discovering his secret internet porn and cybersex habit, something had to give. She desperately hoped that she could motivate him to address the elephant in their bedroom: They had sex about as often as it snowed in their suburban Dallas neighborhood. She walked into their third couple's therapy session on a mission to get Greg and their therapist to agree to make their sex life a priority. It was the least Greg could do after denying her sexual intimacy for most of their nine year marriage.

Greg was having a rather painful experience of his own: Not only did his wife now know what he'd been doing all those nights after she went to bed, but she now wanted him to commit to the one thing that scared him the most, being sexual with her. He was experiencing a double hit of shame: He was ashamed of his secret life and ashamed of failing to be the lover his wife needed. In a perfect world he would love to have a good sex life with Diane, and he found her quite attractive. But in HIS world, the fear of letting her down sexually always displaced this desire. He knew how disappointed she had been with his inability to control his ejaculation and his undependable erections. While he understood Diane's sexual dissatisfaction, he felt paralyzed by the thought of actually doing anything about it.

Diane had never experienced such indifference to her before. From the time she was in high school, guys found her attractive. Her biggest problem had been getting boys to keep their hands to themselves, including Greg, when they were dating. What changed after they got married? As far as she knew, she had had not become *less* attractive. She still received lots of unwanted attention from other men. Why did the man she wanted *most* to show affection seem so disinterested?

1. Stages of Recovery

As much as Diane is ready to address the sexual intimacy deficit in their marriage, the message that she and Greg need to hear is, "First things first." The first thing we do with patients is to help them evaluate and understand where they are along the "Stages of Recovery" as articulated by Dr. Patrick Carnes.[8] They typically have already passed through most of the denial associated with pre-recovery, and have experienced the clarity and resolve that comes with the *Crisis/Decision Stage*, where people realize, "I can't keep living like this, not even for one more day."

In the *Shock Stage*, the reality of how bad things have gotten hits home for both individuals in the relationship. This tends to last up to eight months. It's as if an opaque film of denial on your glasses has been removed and you now can see clearly the extent of the damage done to your relationship, to yourselves, to your finances, to your careers, to your relationships with your children and even to your children's futures. This is where Greg might allow himself to face up to the reality that he would be further ahead in his career if he hadn't been taking so much time maintaining online relationships and staying up late at night looking at porn. Diane might realize how difficult it will be to trust him again. She might also make the connection that Greg's addiction had taken precedence over meeting his responsibilities for the family's financial security.

In the *Grief Stage*, people experience a greater awareness and understanding of losses and pain *throughout their lives*: Spouses typically see how the addict's behavior fits the larger patterns of grief and loss in their own lives, while addicts typically see how the pain they have put others and themselves through fits larger patterns of pain and loss in their own lives. Thus, Diane might see the similarities between how she is feeling abandoned by Greg and how she often felt overlooked in her family of origin. She might remember that her father also seemed to under-perform professionally and had an affair when she was a teenager. Greg might realize that he has been handling his roles of father and husband much like he saw his own father, who left the family for another woman when Greg was in third grade, handle those roles. Both Greg and Diane might use these realizations to deepen their commitments to their personal and couples recovery. Breaking free of their generational dysfunctions and creating new personal legacies will benefit not only themselves but their children as well.

The *Repair Stage* is where both people begin to reconstruct how they understand and feel about themselves and interact with others. There is a major shift from living in contradiction with one's core values to living in alignment with one's integrity. As this shift occurs, people often realize how much they enjoy living authentically. For this to be possible, each person will have needed to work a diligent personal program of recovery to move into the *Repair stage*. Like the *Shock* and *Grief* stages, the *Repair stage* is experienced after a significant amount of proactive, recovery-based work.

The final Stage of recovery is the *Growth Stage*. In this stage, people enjoy the rewards of their recovery efforts. They are thankful for many things in their lives, even including the addiction. Many people recognize that without, it, they probably would not have developed new relationships with themselves and others. They recognize how resilient they have become, which often stands in sharp contrast to how they once felt victimized. Living in *Growth* becomes a renewable energy source that builds on its own abundance.

It is common for some overlap of the stages. Viewed as a pie chart (Figure 3), we see Greg's and Diane's stages of recovery at four months after discovery:

Stages of Recovery

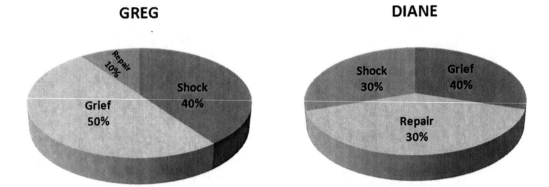

GREG   **DIANE**

For a couple to be good candidates for the SRT Program, both spouses *must* include the Repair Stage in their mix of stages.

2. Addiction and Trauma Work

While working with couples new to recovery, a temptation is to treat the relational problems first, for these are most obvious. Problematic issues typically include: poor communication, finances, lack of time together, parenting conflicts, and all kinds of sexual complaints. Often the couple wants help deciding if they should stay together or end the relationship. However, moving the relational problems and decisions to the top of the treatment pecking order is like trying to build a beautiful new home with no foundation. We certainly acknowledge these relational problems as valid, but emphasize that the time will come to address them directly. In the spirit of "first things first," we need to make sure each person's "house" has a solid foundation, before placing on the roof.

When addictions are present (including Codependence), we treat them first. Greg's internet porn and cybersex addiction needs to be treated. Once he establishes consistent sobriety and has embraced recovery, he will be able to work more efficiently on his core issues, (like how he esteems himself, his boundary practices, and how he is able to be honest and diplomatic with others). He would have a therapist work closely with him while assessing these and other dimensions. At this point he would be in a position to do some trauma work. Trauma work[5] involves examining how he was wounded as a child (in either obvious or subtle ways) and how he behaved as an adult through these early wounds. Wounds can occur when a child experiences overt abuse;

---

[5] The *Story of Our Lives* exercise in Chapter 3 is not designed to replace trauma work done in a therapist's office, but can be adequate for some couples to move forward through the SRT program.

(e.g. physical, or sexual abuse), or covert abuse (e.g. forms of abandonment, neglect or enmeshment).[9]

While Greg may be an obvious candidate for a program of self-assessment and healing, Diane also deserves a healing process. Her history may differ from Greg's, but her wounds and core issues also need understanding and healing. Diane's challenge is to look within, while still coming to terms with the reality of her relationship with Greg. Diane is encouraged in treatment to engage two difficult processes in succession. First, she would be asked to connect with her pain and learn from it. She may gain clarity and strength from the pain. It may empower her to establish her conditions to be in the relationship with Greg. For example, she may state that it is not acceptable for him to be on the computer after she goes to bed or that he needs a blocking filter on the computer, and he must to go to meetings and get a sponsor. These conditions are not expressed so that she may control Greg, but as a clear communication regarding what she needs to feel more safe moving forward.

When she and her therapist agree that the timing is right, she will also consider how she participated in the dysfunctional aspects of their relationship. While stopping short of taking responsibility for Greg's acting out, she needs to search within for answers to questions like; "What have I been doing that has not been beneficial to our relationship? Have I been enabling, critical, controlling or avoiding? Have I asked directly for things I need or want?"

Dianne needs to be working on a parallel path with Greg, by looking at her core issues and how they evolved from her trauma history Both Diane and Greg must develop an understanding about how they were dysfunctional with each other; about how they were relating through their wounds, or operating from childlike states. Then additional criteria can be used to determine if they are ready to begin the work of healing together, using SRT. They do not need to have it ALL figured out. They simply need to understand how they have been dysfunctional, both from an individual and relational standpoint.

Figure 4:

How We Got Here

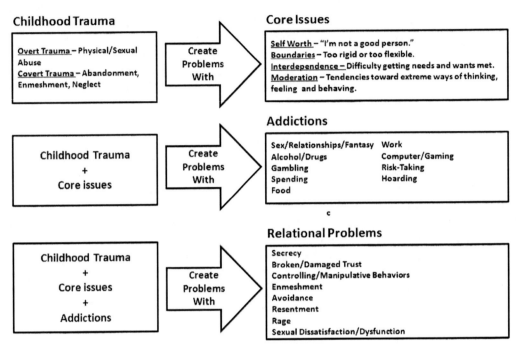

Childhood Trauma

<u>Overt Trauma</u> – Physical/Sexual Abuse
<u>Covert Trauma</u> – Abandonment, Enmeshment, Neglect

Create Problems With

Core Issues

<u>Self Worth</u> – "I'm not a good person."
<u>Boundaries</u> – Too rigid or too flexible.
<u>Interdependence</u> – Difficulty getting needs and wants met.
<u>Moderation</u> – Tendencies toward extreme ways of thinking, feeling and behaving.

**Childhood Trauma
+
Core issues**

Create Problems With

Addictions

Sex/Relationships/Fantasy   Work
Alcohol/Drugs   Computer/Gaming
Gambling   Risk-Taking
Spending   Hoarding
Food

**Childhood Trauma
+
Core issues
+
Addictions**

Create Problems With

Relational Problems

Secrecy
Broken/Damaged Trust
Controlling/Manipulative Behaviors
Enmeshment
Avoidance
Resentment
Rage
Sexual Dissatisfaction/Dysfunction

Adapted from Pia Mellody

Other couples have a different dynamic. Early in their treatment, Phillip and Renee reported that Phillip turned to internet porn and massage parlors because he was feeling sexually rejected by Renee. Renee was devastated to learn about his acting out behaviors, and felt a tremendous amount of guilt. She knew she had failed to be the lover her husband needed and deserved. She found herself getting angry and feeling hurt, but would quickly realize that if she had been more available, he would have been less tempted to look elsewhere to satisfy his sexual needs. Phillip reinforced this perspective whenever they discussed what had been happening. When they arrived at their first therapy appointment, their shared goal was to have more sex. They agreed that to reach this goal, Renee needed to learn why she did not have sexual desire and what she could do to change.

Hopefully, Renee and Phillip find a therapist who appreciates their main motivations for beginning treatment, but who also understands that it would be inappropriate to focus on sparking their sex life right off the bat. Their individual and shared sexuality are undeniably valid therapy issues. However, Renee and Phillip, like most couples, would be best served by first examining their family of origin trauma histories, core issues, and how the trauma and core issues created the breeding ground for addiction and codependence. As all three factors (trauma, core issues and addiction) are being addressed, the dysfunction in their relationship will be understood more completely than their original assertions that pointed only to sexual symptoms and struggles. Then it will be much easier to directly address the very sexual issues that motivated them to seek treatment.

One way of understanding the purpose of addictions, sexual and otherwise, is that they are *stabilizing agents*.[10] They emerge and take hold so that they may support us under the weight of shame and feelings of inadequacy and external stress. While acting out almost always delivers on the short-term promise of escape, a steep price is paid for this temporary relief: Not only do the original sources of the uncomfortable feelings remain, but the acting out behavior is never free and clear of consequences.

In recovery, when acting out behaviors are deliberately set aside, we trade short-term temporary relief for the freedom that comes with living in reality, even if it is a painful reality. One of the ongoing challenges of recovery is experiencing our inner worlds as never before. We *feel* our feelings because we are no longer self-medicating the pain away. Self-medicating behaviors apply to *all* addictions including food, spending, gambling, overwork, over-exercising and co-addiction.

When these feelings are felt in new and powerful ways, there needs to be enough recovery in place to tolerate them and to have a mature experience with them. Otherwise, there is a risk of jumping from one addiction to another. For example, recovering sex addicts may turn to obsessive exercise or overwork or overeating when they stop acting out sexually. All of these factors indicate a need to approach couples recovery carefully. When a couple's SRT treatment begins prematurely, there is a strong likelihood that the treatment will fail and reinforce doubts about continuing the relationship. We believe that one of the therapist's main responsibilities is setting couples up for success by developing a treatment plan that has a properly ordered series of focus areas and action steps.

The first priority always involves aggressively treating addictions and codependence. Only then is it possible to focus squarely on individual trauma, personal core issues, and couples recovery tasks (e.g. Formal Disclosure). *Then* you are positioned to work on intimacy, where each of you is asked to renew your commitment to the other. The intimacy work is actually the final stage of couples healing, but it is often the case that couples want to begin treatment here. In other scenarios, one spouse gets "left behind" in early treatment, as the other spouse gets most of their treatment resources and focus.

What we help couples cultivate is a spirit and practice of partnership and collaboration. One *half* of a couple in recovery does not equal partnership and collaboration, yet this is all too familiar for many. The SRT program clearly works best when: a) each of you has embraced your own recovery from addiction/codependence and b) when each of you has pursued healing around trauma and has addressed core issues. Thus, on each side there is a growing understanding and integration of boundaries, an appropriate connection with self-esteem, an ability to be real and diplomatic with each other, and growing abilities to exercise good self-care and live in moderation.

3. Formal Disclosure

In addition to requiring that each spouse comes to the SRT Program with an adequate amount of recovery from addictions and trauma, the couple also must complete a full and comprehensive disclosure prior to beginning SRT. A disclosure is when the addict and partner, with guidance from their therapist, plan a formal meeting in which the addict reads a thoroughly prepared statement listing all acting out behaviors. The main purpose of this meeting is to help the spouse feel more secure with the idea that the addict is now committed to being truthful, despite whatever history of secrecy existed to maintain the addictive behavior(s). Given the difficult nature of this exercise, it also gives the addict a real test regarding his/her commitment to rigorous honesty. The spouse needs to be involved in planning the disclosure so that s/he has a voice relative to: a) what s/he hopes to gain from the disclosure process, b) what concerns s/he has about the disclosure process, c) the level of detail to be shared. It can also be helpful to review the spouse's previous experiences with asking the addict for the truth. Often, the spouse received information in a piece-meal ("drip-drip") manner, which always undermines trust. The disclosure is intended to honor the spouse by telling the whole truth, so there will be no unpleasant surprises to discover later. It is also a time for the spouse to ask any questions that s/he has been holding back or to inquire further about anything heard during the disclosure. Nothing is asked of the spouse during the meeting. The planning and preparation for this very important process, as well as the disclosure meeting itself, is best done with the guidance of a Certified Sex Addiction Therapist (CSAT).[6]

4. Emotional Restitution

Another component required before beginning SRT is *Emotional Restitution.*[11] Like a formal disclosure, an emotional restitution process requires a significant amount of reflection and planning. It asks the addict to go beyond simply listing *what happened* while acting out, but to also take responsibility for the deception, manipulation and exploitation that went on as the addict took advantage of the spouse's positive traits. A prepared statement called a *Clarification Letter*[7] is carefully drafted by the addict and read to the spouse during a meeting dedicated to this purpose. There is nothing asked of the spouse during this meeting (such as forgiveness). The spouse has the option to ask for clarification regarding any content or may ask any questions about the themes being addressed. Emotional restitution also can be a tremendously powerful way to help addicts generate and connect with real feelings of empathy for their spouses.

After the addict's emotional restitution, the spouse may be in a better position to reflect on his/her contributions to the dysfunctions in the relationship. This can be shared with the addict during a subsequent meeting. This mutual process of taking personal responsibility reinforces to the spouse that s/he gets strength from his or her *own* recovery and not just from the spouse's recovery. This attitude greatly enhances

---

[6] For the most complete resource on the process of disclosure, we recommend *Disclosing Secrets* by Deborah Corley and Jennifer Schneider.

[7] There is an entire section on Clarification Letters written by Ken Wells in the *Recovery Start Kit* (see Bibliography).

the likelihood of a successful recovery for the couple. It is best described by the Recovering Couples Anonymous (RCA) analogy of the three-legged stool approach to couples healing: One leg is "My Recovery," one is "Your Recovery," and the last is "Our Recovery." This attitude greatly enhances the likelihood of a successful recovery for the couple and sets the stage for a successful SRT experience.

5. Review of Critical Incidents of Betrayal

Even after all of these steps have been taken, the spouse's feelings of deep pain and anger may still continue. It is also not uncommon for him/her to be seen as being difficult or uncompromising by the addict and even by some therapists. However, trauma and addiction expert Dr. Kenneth Adams has developed a model that honors the spouse's ongoing pain: Rather than blaming the spouse, his model encourages revisiting some of the most painful incidents of betrayal that have been especially devastating to the partner or spouse.[12] The rationale for this is that the betrayals themselves have created trauma for the spouse. Trauma is not automatically resolved by even the most thorough disclosure and emotional restitution. As helpful as those instruments are, one or more of these betrayals may need to be revisited in order to help the spouse achieve the healing that would allow him/her to continue to reinvest in the relationship.

In Dr. Adams' model, the spouse is given an opportunity to list, state and discuss the *most* hurtful experiences, how s/he was affected back then, and the ongoing effects after learning of the betrayals. The addict is asked to listen respectfully and to express whatever genuine empathy s/he has. The process of reviewing these critical incidents of betrayal has the effect of validating the spouse's experience. It also allows the addict to be more relational by experiencing negative affect from the spouse and then honoring it with an empathic response. The entire process is intimacy enhancing because of the mutual vulnerability involved.

***

When spouses and partners have met the above criteria for readiness, it is important that they think seriously about the kind of sexual intimacy they would like to enjoy. With this in mind, the next chapter presents a framework for understanding and embracing a sexual intimacy grounded in recovery and emotional intimacy.

5

What IS Healthy Sexuality?

The mystery surrounding how to define, understand and approach healthy sexuality has confused and confounded many couples in recovery. In early recovery, much energy and focus is placed on avoiding *unhealthy* sexual behaviors and patterns. With a certain amount of abstinence from those behaviors as well as other recovery achievements (see Ch 4 "Timing is Everything"), a couple has a fresh opportunity to answer for themselves the question: *What is Healthy Sexuality?*

There are many answers to this question in books, research articles, seminars, talk-shows and magazines. It would seem difficult to discern the correct answer, even if there were such a thing! Instead of debating the merits of the multitude of varying opinions, we present in this chapter the philosophy and vision of healthy sexuality that makes the most sense to us and works best for our recovering patients. This philosophy allows for the proactive, healthy sexual behaviors and attitudes that will characterize the new and vastly improved version of your individual and shared sexuality. At stake is a tremendous opportunity to heal and grow both personally and relationally. The basis of SRT is a belief that *it is possible to identify and bid farewell to old, unhealthy ways of thinking, feeling and acting sexually, and to deliberately choose new, functional ways that can be integrated into your very being.* This chapter provides the foundational basis for the Planned Intimate Experiences found in Part II of this book.

Why We Must Talk About This In Recovery

While a more comfortable path might avoid discussing so directly the delicate and damaged fabric of your sexual intimacy, there is a very simple reason why that path will not serve your long-term interests: Your sexual thoughts, feelings and behaviors *have been affected by the addiction,* regardless of whether you have a specific sexual barrier or dissatisfaction right now. Some effects are obvious, such as the pain felt from the addict's sexual acting out behavior. Spouses suffer such a blow from the disclosure or discovery of the addictive behavior. Their ability to trust is severely damaged, and for many this makes it impossible to be sexually intimate for some time. On the other hand, disclosure and discovery can trigger some spouses into a *hyper*sexual state. This is in response to feeling responsible and inadequate to meet the addict's sexual needs. They become more sexually available than ever, attempting to eliminate the addict's temptation to get those needs met outside the relationship.

Some of the effects of addiction on sexuality are more subtle, like the tolerance to stimulation and the craving for intensity that the addict's brain develops from repeated exposure to internet pornography or risk-taking acting-out behavior. There is no way for intimacy-based sex with one's spouse to compete with the intensity and stimulation of cybersex, internet porn and other forms of acting out. At some point most spouses reach this conclusion, and many question whether they will ever be enough to satisfy their spouse. Furthermore, sex addicts typically possess a relatively naïve or adolescent awareness of how to experience a healthy, mutually satisfying sex life in a committed relationship. For all the sexual activity in which they have engaged, their sexual knowledge is often underdeveloped. Many sex addicts have a frame of reference about what is sexually pleasurable to others based on what they have seen in pornography or what they find in sexual chat rooms, blogs, or in their adrenaline-driven adulterous encounters.

Often it seems there is so much sexual wreckage to clean up, it will never get done. However, the fact is that countless couples have used the pain of their sexual brokenness to guide them toward seeking the special healing that their relationship needs. *SRT can help you to do just that by providing a framework in which you can connect with your sexual, emotional and spiritual selves, and intentionally decide how to be in relationship with each other through all of these dimensions of intimacy.* Ironically, the opportunity to achieve healing in this most important area may have not been realized without the discovery or disclosure of the compulsive sexual behavior. Appreciation for this irony is usually the result of much time and effort in recovery, and it can be very helpful to couples in finding meaning for their suffering and redemption for their pain.

When addiction is present, the damage extends to everyone touched by it. In the case of sex addicts and spouses, the damage is more challenging because your sexual selves as well as your shared sexuality cannot be avoided. Even in situations where couples mutually agree to a period of celibacy, it is intended to be just that: a *period* (usually 60-90 days). This means that if your relationship continues, you must necessarily revisit a significant amount of uncomfortable territory.

For this reason, many sexual paradigm shifts need to occur for anyone involved in a relationship that has existed in the environment of addiction. Dr. Patrick Carnes writes,

> "Central to the paradigm shift will be a new understanding of their sexuality. They will learn to see sex as an authentic expression of self that can be safe and loving. They will also…combine intimacy with sex. They will discover sex actually works best when there is healthy bonding."[13]

Two of the most significant paradigm shifts addressed in this chapter involve:
1. Shifting from sex as an activity that occurs in isolation to one which occurs in intimacy.
2. Shifting from sex as an activity that pursues intensity, control or escape to one which welcomes pleasure while being present and free of demands or expectations.

The Big Picture: Healthy Sexuality Begins with a Healthy Self

It is entirely possible to achieve these shifts, but many people in recovery wonder exactly *how* to move in the direction of healthy sexuality. It can seem like a case of "good-news, bad news." The good news is that we live in an era with more material available on sexual satisfaction than ever. The bad news is *also* that we live in an era with more material on sexual satisfaction than ever. The available menu of behavioral techniques intended to increase sexual satisfaction is seemingly endless. It can be found in thousands of websites and in magazines at checkout stands of every grocery store. You can spend a lifetime picking and choosing from this menu hoping that the next variation, trick or technique is the key to a satisfying sex life. You might even find that some of the items actually work because you may reach a higher level of arousal or enjoy more sexual frequency than usual.

For couples in stable marriages where both spouses are experiencing a satisfying sex life, picking items from this menu in an effort to spice things up can be a fine thing to try. Yet, for couples in recovery from sexual addiction, a much more comprehensive approach to establishing a healthy, mutually satisfying sexuality is required. This is because the damage done to sexuality by addiction has created a fresh trauma. Furthermore, each spouse's unresolved trauma issues (see Chapter 3 *"Story of My Life"*) likely have been triggered, compounding the challenge.

When this is the case any new "hot sex" techniques, on their own, are likely to yield only short-term gains, if any. Couples usually find themselves circling back to their familiar frustrations as they continue to interact through well-worn patterns grounded in unresolved trauma. The following story of Angela and Dylan illustrates many typical challenges faced in couples sexual recovery. Fortunately, both Angela and Dylan were willing to explore their personal histories to make sense of how things could have gone so far off-track. As this chapter continues, we will review some of the healing they experienced through the insights they developed.

For the last seven years of their 12 year marriage, Dylan had been addicted to amateur porn sites. He found them to be incredibly arousing because the amateur couples looked so normal, "not like vamped-up, beefed-up porn stars." He often secretly masturbated to these videos after Angela had gone to bed. Early in his treatment, his perception was that he was making a lot of changes, especially giving up porn, yet he could see no willingness on Angela's part to address his biggest source of frustration: their sex life. Dylan was very clear that it wasn't so much the frequency with which they had sex (about once a week) that he found insufficient, but the lack of willingness on Angela's part to try anything new. During our first session Dylan said:

> "We always do the same old things, except on my birthday. That's when I get about 2 minutes of oral sex and THEN we go back to the same old things. I don't think we have tried more than four positions in the past 12 years. It's always the same; the same days of the week, same times of day, same silence from her, same steps from point A to B to her orgasm to intercourse. I have read a lot of books about what turns women on, but she doesn't want anything but vanilla sex. So now I have all this useless knowledge! And I've given her books to read on

41

what turns men on in bed, but I don't think she's read a single page- that hurts me, it really does. It pretty much confirms what I already knew, that she doesn't really care enough to try something new that is really important to me. And sex has *always* been really important to me- she knew that before we got married! Looking back, I guess the best sex we had was before we got married. Then something changed and she just lost interest a few months after the wedding. I call it "Angela's False Advertisement."

Damage Assessment

The story of Angela and Dylan highlights the damage from addiction. In online pornography, Dylan found reinforcement of his belief that Angela was less sexual than most women, which also reinforced him feeling like her victim. He cycled through feeling rejected by her and then feeling entitled to have the vicarious experience of an intense and edgy sex life through the couples in the videos he watched. Here is Angela's story:

"I felt his resentment long before the addiction came to light. There were times when he looked at me like I was his mortal enemy. Other times, he ignored me as if I wasn't even in the room. When we had sex, it felt rushed, driven, and sometimes even angry. He always needed to know if I had an orgasm. Sometimes I got the feeling that he was connecting more with my breasts and genitals than with *me*.

I will always remember the shock of opening his laptop on that awful afternoon and finding it filled with pornographic videos and images. It was as if everything instantly made sense, but in the worst possible way. Of course he would look to this stuff, because he was so obviously unhappy with what I enjoyed (or used to enjoy) sexually. It kind of harshly confirmed what I already suspected: I just wasn't enough for him. As I sit here right now, I can't imagine ever getting those images out of my mind. The women were all about 15 years younger than me and had bodies like I will never have. And I guess now I know what he wants sex to be like for us. They were doing the kind of things that Dylan has been asking me to do, like having sex in front of their windows, in their cars, in public restrooms, even anal sex- something I will never agree to! If this is what he needs to get aroused, then it's no wonder he's been having trouble with erections lately."

As a result of how harmful the sexually addictive behaviors were to both Dylan and Angela, their healing process involved jumping through some challenging hoops. Dylan needed help confronting his sense of being Angela's victim as well as his skewed sense of sexual norms and his sense of entitlement. Angela had symptoms of Post-Traumatic Stress Disorder, such as intrusive thoughts and flashbacks to what she had seen on his computer. She needed help with her fear that she might never be able to let Dylan see her naked again, let alone be sexual with him.

With great effort and strong support, Dylan was able to make significant progress in treatment. For example, he was willing to embrace the process of Emotional Restitution, taking full responsibility for his acting out behaviors and the pain Angela experienced from discovering it. He owned responsibility for how critical and demanding he had been of her sexually, and how he manipulated her with his pouting and anger. He acknowledged that his chronic criticism created distance between them and managed his fear of close relationships. Finally, he promised to be patient with Angela as she tried to cope with her feelings of sadness, grief, fear and anger.

On her side, Angela gave herself permission to share the burden of her pain with a 12- Step group for recovering spouses and partners of sex addicts. She also let the pain that she was feeling guide her in discerning what types of boundaries she needed to stay in relationship with Dylan. With the backing of her support network, she formulated a list of conditions (a "Safety List") she needed Dylan to honor. If he failed to keep up his end of the deal, she told him, she would have a difficult time remaining in the relationship. This was not delivered as a threat or power play. It was simply Angela's truth and that was the spirit in which she shared it. None of their proactive steps *erased* the damage, but each was a significant component of their personal and shared healing. Finally, both were willing to examine their personal histories to try to make sense of their unhappiness.

Healthy Sexuality is INTIMACY-based

One of the great paradigm shifts that occur during SRT involves discovering the joy and freedom of intimacy-based sexuality. We use the term "Functional Sexuality" because it represents the opposite of dysfunctional sexuality. An ongoing task for any recovering couple is to discover how a functional, interdependent sexual intimacy can grow out of a functional, interdependent *emotional* intimacy. The following figure illustrates the continuum that exists around interdependence. [8]

---

[8] Adapted from Pia Mellody

Figure 5:

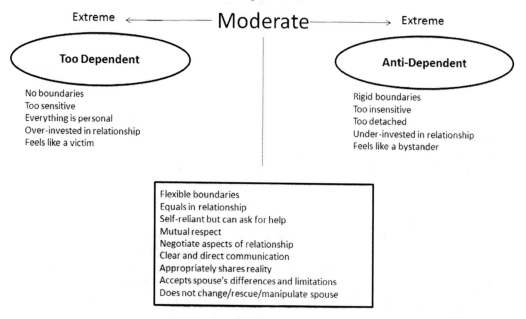

Interdependence

Extreme ←——————— Moderate ———————→ Extreme

Too Dependent

No boundaries
Too sensitive
Everything is personal
Over-invested in relationship
Feels like a victim

Anti-Dependent

Rigid boundaries
Too insensitive
Too detached
Under-invested in relationship
Feels like a bystander

Flexible boundaries
Equals in relationship
Self-reliant but can ask for help
Mutual respect
Negotiate aspects of relationship
Clear and direct communication
Appropriately shares reality
Accepts spouse's differences and limitations
Does not change/rescue/manipulate spouse

Functional Sexuality involves three concepts:
  a) *Mutual Commitment*
  b) *Embracing self-worth*
  c) *Communicating sexual realities* (desires, wants, curiosities, comforts, discomforts, limits) *while practicing functional boundaries.*

The Components of Functional Sexuality:
Mutual Commitment

Because sexuality can be experienced in many different contexts, there is a distinction to be made between sexuality in non-committed relationships and in mutually committed relationships. The fact is that much more is required of each person's capacity for intimacy in order to experience functional sexuality in a committed relationship. Being sexual in non-committed relationships does not require much at all. For example, there are websites with *millions* of openly married subscribers looking to meet other married subscribers for everything from a "quickie" to an ongoing sexual relationship, with no strings attached. In addition, there is a robust community that practices pain-exchange sex (BDSM) and believes that anything goes, as long as it's consensual. Many people can be sexually satisfied in casual "hook-ups" or have intensely pleasurable, high-intensity sex with themselves and others, only to struggle with low desire, low arousal and other sexual dysfunctions in committed relationships.

Functional sexual intimacy is not an intensity-seeking, performance evaluating, athletic event like Dylan may have envisioned. On the contrary, it has a uniquely felt sense to it that can only be experienced if two components are in place: a sense of *inherent worth* and *functional boundaries*. These are components that a vast majority of pre-recovery addicts and their spouses have little experience with.

Inherent Worth

When you possess a functional and healthy sense of your inherent worth, you are able to esteem yourself from within. While it might feel good to receive compliments, affirmation and positive feedback from your spouse, you are not *dependent* on external reinforcement to feel good about yourself. This becomes especially important as it relates to your sexual relationship. Both of you can develop a positive sexual self-image in which you are able to affirm your sexual selves. For example, you can gradually build experiences that reinforce your sense of being worthy of a nurturing, pleasurable, loving sexual relationship.

This is in contrast to Dylan's typical automatic interpretations when Angela was not comfortable with his ideas to "spice things up." He would tell himself that Angela didn't love him; that Angela didn't value or respect what was important to him; or that something was wrong with Angela for not being open or interested in trying something new. We understand such negative, automatic interpretations as being trauma-based repetitions of old, deeply ingrained messages learned in childhood. They have a very detrimental effect on our adult relationship satisfaction and often enable victim thinking. The antidote is to replace them with a more functional, reality-based interpretation. This is the desired outcome of the hard work of recovery which is reinforced and refined in the SRT program.

Dylan's recovery is a good example. As he embraced the challenge to understand why he had made the interpretations he had, he recognized parts of his personal history that helped him make sense of things. First, when he and his therapist reviewed his family of origin, he identified strongly with a "hero" role in his family. He was put on a pedestal for his appearance and maturity as well as his academic performance and athletic accomplishments. He relished the praise from his parents, teachers, and coaches. He was rewarded with new toys and money for getting straight A's or for making an All-Star team. But the best payoffs were the *surprises* his parents would give him that he had not requested. Those were fantastic. Over time, he received the latest computer games, tickets to sold-out concerts, and a new car for getting a scholarship to an Ivy League school. With treatment, he came to understand how he had learned that his self worth was closely tied to his performance and to what he received from others. The highest form of validation of his worth was when others would do something new, different and better than ever for him in recognition of his excellent performance.

In treatment, he looked at his relationship history. He knew from the time he was 15, that girls found him attractive, but he always felt insecure. He had a nagging feeling that he had to win his girlfriends over with his impressive achievements, quick wit, and his patented ability to get a girl's parents to really like him. Although his family and church were strongly opposed to pre-marital sex, Dylan missed no opportunities to act on his sexual feelings as a teen. When he started to be sexual with his girlfriends, he discovered a feeling so powerfully validating that it was even better than his new car. He would do almost anything to get his dates to have sex so he could experience the rush of validation as well as a restored sense of security in the relationship. He felt most secure and validated when his girlfriend was willing to be sexual, despite risk of getting caught. When a girlfriend declined his advances, it was like a hole opened up inside. He would feel devastated and would not try to hide his frustration. Many relationships ended because Dylan's girlfriends grew tired of the cycle of being pressured and manipulated sexually.

Dylan developed an understanding of how much he needed "other-esteem" in order to feel *any* sense of worth. The highest form of "other-esteem" was delivered when women would push the envelope sexually with him. He reflected in his therapist's office: "I can see now that I was going to be this way no matter who I married. But Angela was probably the only woman who would put up with my sexual pressure for this long. I made her out to be the reason for my unhappiness but it was really all my old crap." His newfound compassion gave their relationship a new chance to heal.

During Dylan's treatment, he was able to achieve a significant paradigm shift: For the first time, he accepted that he is precious and loveable *just because he exists,* regardless of what others thought of him (or would do with him). He was able to recognize others as equal to him in value, even when they had needs and wants that were at odds with his own. This was especially important in his relationship with Angela: As he stopped going "one-up" on her, they gradually developed a sense of partnership in creating their sexuality together.

Consequently, Dylan's new interpretations when Angela declined his sexual requests were characterized by acceptance of and respect for her preferences. Dylan realized how much less intensity he had around their sex life, and recognized this difference as a welcome change from the "old way." Their sex life was not so high stakes anymore because he did not *need it* to feel good about himself. He worked to keep his newfound perspectives about himself and his interactions with Angela as conscious as possible, because he knew how easy it would be to slip back into his default mode. Rather than feeling dependent on Angela for a sense of security (and then resentful when she "failed" to do so) he was more connected than ever with his own ability to make himself feel secure.

Functional Boundaries: Sharing with a Safety Net

As important and valuable as it is to share sexual realities with each other, we do not advocate that you merely resolve to start sharing more authentically with each other. Sharing needs to be safe, with a *functional boundary system*[9] in place, to regulate the experience and flow of our perceptions and feelings. It certainly helps to have a partner who is able to consistently operate within the same functional boundaries.

For example, Angela might become aware that she would like a different kind of touch or a different progression of touch. If she is operating from a perspective that

---

[9] You will be asked to review Appendix A, which contains Pia Mellody's model of Functional Boundaries, before beginning the SRT Program.

both she and Dylan have inherent worth and she is using her functional boundaries, she could state her reality to him as follows. "Dylan, I really like it when you rub my back. Do you think you could try a softer touch? I would really like that." Contrast this with a boundary-less approach that does not imply inherent worth for either: "Dylan! How many times do I have to tell you to use a lighter touch? It's like talking to the wall!"

Dylan realized that before treatment he had been engaging in blame, manipulation, and intensity with his sexual requests. In response, Angela had experienced shame, guilt, fear, and anger. Many times, she would agree to be sexual despite not wanting to. In effect, she was not giving full consent as much as she was being coerced into being sexual. Angela could not enjoy those times because she was merely catering to Dylan's desires. Dylan could not enjoy those times because he could *tell* that Angela was merely catering to his desires. Angela could not find her own sexual desire because Dylan's seemed so overwhelming. It did not help matters when Angela was subjected to Dylan's ongoing sexual critiques and complaints.

In treatment, Dylan and Angela learned how practicing functional boundaries promotes respectful communication of sexual availability and preferences. Angela learned to respect herself when she was unavailable by clearly communicating her reality to Dylan. At those times she would say something like, "I'm sorry I'm not available for that right now. I think tomorrow would be better. That way, we'll have more time and I'll have more energy than I do right now. How would that be for you?" Dylan respected Angela by not taking her "no" personally. This gave her room to say "yes" to another time and to mean it. This is the basis of mutual consent. It is when both spouses feel free to be authentic, whether it is saying "no" without fear of consequence or "yes" with enthusiasm.

When each of you is connecting with your inherent worth, identifying your sexual realities, and sharing them while practicing functional boundaries, it is highly likely that you will enjoy a *much richer sexual intimacy than ever before*. In fact, this is exactly what we expect by the time you are about halfway through the SRT program. When at one time the question may have been, "How much *worse* can this get?" the new question may be, "How *good* can this get?"

The Circulation Model

The answer depends on how you are able to nurture your intimacy inside and outside the bedroom. We think of this as a "Circulation Model." When the circulation is flowing properly, each "room" benefits from the positively charged atmosphere in the other room, creating a positive feedback loop.

Figure 6: [10]

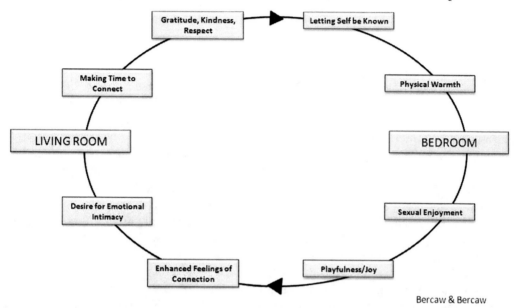

Circulation Model of Sexual Intimacy

Gratitude, Kindness, Respect

Letting Self be Known

Making Time to Connect

Physical Warmth

LIVING ROOM

BEDROOM

Desire for Emotional Intimacy

Sexual Enjoyment

Enhanced Feelings of Connection

Playfulness/Joy

Bercaw & Bercaw

The idea that you can have good flow in one room without the other is not realistic. Nevertheless, gender stereotypes have traditionally painted a picture where men enjoy sex without needing much of an emotional connection, while women prioritize emotional connection and can do without sex. More recently, it has been viewed as progressive that women can enjoy casual, detached sex as much as men. However, this way of thinking is very similar to the compartmentalized manner in which addicts typically approach sexuality. Even in their committed relationships, many addicts remain sexually disconnected. SRT is designed to promote a truly integrated partnership. *You are integrating emotional connection with erotic experiences to allow the two "rooms" to feed off of the best aspects of each other.*

For example, when you are pursuing pleasure during times of sexual intimacy, the bedroom door is not sealed shut. Rather, the energy from the living room continues to circulate inside the bedroom and vice versa. Thus, you may experience the warm carry-over of your living room connection during your sexual intimacy and the passionate bedroom connection helping you feel more emotionally close while in the living room. In Dylan's case, he learned not to expect Angela to be sexually interested while they were in a state of conflict. Instead, his growth involved appreciating that their best sexual times occurred when they were feeling close and connected. As

---

[10] Graphic adapted from Rosemary Basson's Non-Linear Model of Female Sexual Response

Angela began to reclaim her own sexual feelings, she learned that their positive sexual experiences often enhanced feeling close and connected to Dylan.

The Circulation Model is promoted by the two-track (emotional and sexual) approach of the SRT program. While it emphasizes balance between emotional intimacy and sexual intimacy, it *does not* place a ceiling on sexual pleasure. The hope is that you will find yourselves gradually trending in the direction of what we call *"Sexual Abundance."*

Sexual Abundance

Conventional wisdom and popular culture tells us that the *best* way to increase sexual satisfaction is to break through sexual barriers by engaging in *new sexual activities*. While it is generally accepted that experimenting with new activities (assuming mutual comfort and mutual desire to try them) can add welcomed variety to a couple's sex life, it is not the *only* way, and may not be the *best* way. One problem with the "breaking through barriers" approach is that there are only so many new tricks to be tried. You can vary positions, locations, accessories and risk, but at some point it might occur to you that you have reached the edge of your sexual universe.

But wouldn't it be great if you could live in a sexual universe that had limitless potential, that was renewable, and within your own power to access? Where you could have a new and different experience *in the moment* while engaging in a familiar activity? No new ground would need to be broken in terms of what you are doing, but you would find yourself in new territory because of how you are *experiencing* that particular moment. You would feel a noticeably heightened connection as you enjoy a mutually pleasurable experience with your loved one. So, if it seems like you have tried all the sexual activities you would like to try, that does not have to signify the end of your erotic enjoyment. In fact, if you believe as we do, that each experience differs in some ways from any previous one, this means that you will always be adding new pages to your menu!

The variables that affect the experience of sexual abundance are *intimacy and novelty*. Both are fueled by *freely chosen vulnerability*. When you experience sexual abundance, your sex life, by its very nature, will be have limitless potential to help you experience yourself and your spouse in pleasurable and connecting ways. Sexual abundance *does* involve pursuing your pleasure to the fullest extent. Renowned psychoanalyst and sexuality expert Dr. Michael Bader endorses this perspective as he advocates for each person to "surrender to one's own selfish excitement without guilt or burdensome feelings of responsibility." Of course, he is not using the word 'selfish' in the classic sense of the word, but as a means of emphasizing the importance of being closely *attuned to your own sexual reality* during times of intimacy. In order to do this, it is necessary to let go of so many of the thoughts that guide us in our non-sexual moments of life, such as when we are expected to be neat, quiet, contained, or deferential. Then you are in a position to choose to share your sexual realities with each other. However, all of this is done within the context of respecting each other's boundaries and operating from an equal position.

It may be counterintuitive, but the practice of functional boundaries actually creates a greater sense of freedom to enjoy whatever is happening *right now,* instead of looking too far ahead. SRT encourages you to share your sexual realities in truth and love with your spouse by consistently choosing to make yourself vulnerable. Sharing sexual realities can come in many forms:

- Sharing a *request* such as, "I'm wondering if you might want to shower together later tonight and see what happens?"
- Sharing a *thought*, "The last time we got together was great, but I think I was uncomfortable with how we ended up."
- Asking a *question*, "What was that like for you when I asked you to slow down a little?"
- Sharing a *feeling*, "I had a lot of passion, love and joy about our last time together and I have a lot of gratitude when I think about how far we've come together."
- Taking an *action*, such as showing your spouse how you prefer to be touched or kissed.

Figure 7:

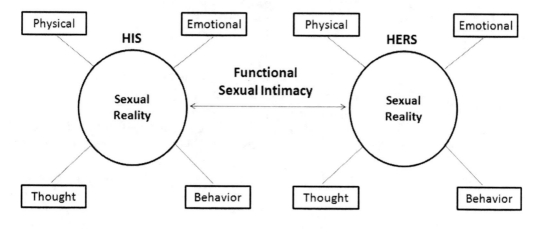

Functional Sexual Intimacy Through Sharing Sexual Realities

Physical   **HIS**   **Emotional**   **Physical**   **HERS**   **Emotional**

Sexual Reality   **Functional Sexual Intimacy**   **Sexual Reality**

Thought   **Behavior**   **Thought**   **Behavior**

**Sharing sexual realities requires the use of the "safety net" of functional boundaries. (See Appendix A)

When you consistently choose vulnerability, you necessarily create a novel moment, and it can be every bit as connecting as actually trying a new sexual activity. What becomes new and different is how you are coming to know yourselves and each other. You each bring your new levels of self-knowledge and the new ways you know each other to your sexually intimate experiences.

As a result you end up with a new experience, even if you are engaging in an "old" activity. Of course, there is nothing wrong with trying new activities. In fact, most of what you will be doing in the SRT program is likely to be new!

<u>s</u>
<u>Figure 8:</u>

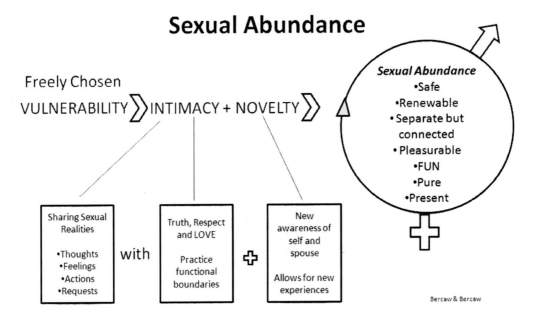

Sexual Abundance

Freely Chosen

VULNERABILITY 》》INTIMACY + NOVELTY 》》

Sexual Abundance
- •Safe
- •Renewable
- • Separate but connected
- • Pleasurable
- •FUN
- •Pure
- •Present

Sharing Sexual Realities

•Thoughts
•Feelings
•Actions
•Requests

with

Truth, Respect and LOVE

Practice functional boundaries

New awareness of self and spouse

Allows for new experiences

Bercaw & Bercaw

Doug and Katrina remarked during their SRT treatment that they noticed kissing felt different. As Katrina said, "It's not like he's doing much differently physically. It's more like I can feel him there with me, like he wants to be kissing me. It's not just kissing to cross off the list so we can move on to the good parts. I can tell he's more interested in me and how I'm enjoying the kiss. It's like we are kissing for the first time!"

Doug was also aware of the differences: "In the past, I didn't think much about the kissing part. It was more of a stepping stone to what would come next. But it really helped to be able to hear how much Katrina would like to enjoy kissing more; she put herself out there a little bit and I respect that. I'm realizing that I've been missing out on the pleasure of kissing. I just didn't know it. Now I feel like I'm kissing the girl I'm dating as much as the woman I've been married to for 22 years."

As you experience sexual abundance, you may have some thoughts like these:

"I never knew before that I could ask for what I wanted."
"I never knew what it was like to be so present and connected with her during sex."
"I never knew he was so worried about disappointing me."
"I never knew she *had* any sexual preferences."

51

The fact is that you don't *need* to become an expert in the Kama Sutra. You need to become an expert in knowing your true self and deliberately choosing how to share it. We encourage you to connect with the following vision and to recall it as part of your daily spiritual practice:

As you work your way through the SRT program, you will naturally be guided in the direction of Sexual Abundance through the Planned Intimate Experiences. You will gradually become more comfortable choosing to share your evolving realities with each other. You will experience the powerful connecting potential of mutually chosen vulnerability within the safety of functional boundaries. You will recognize that choosing to be mutually vulnerable is a renewable and sustainable source of energy in your relationship. Because of your ability to access this relational energy, you will find a new quality to your experience of even familiar activities. You may also be more open to trying some things that you haven't tried before because now you feel more safety and trust with each other. The circulation between your living room and your bedroom will gain strength and momentum, as each feeds off of the positive energy from the other. You will make the wonderful shift from experiencing sexuality in the restricted grasp of addiction to experiencing your newly claimed sexuality in the abundance of recovery.

6

Barriers to Treatment

There are several potential obstacles that can complicate any couple's successful progress through SRT. Each can be overcome.

1. "But Things are Better Now"

One of the paradoxes in recovery is that when some relief from longstanding problems is finally achieved, it is often necessary to delve *deeper* into the problems. The fact is that by the time a couple has met the criteria to be ready to begin SRT, each spouse usually reports that their relationship is better now than before recovery. Some spouses reflect on this discovery and think, "Do we really need to do all this when things are so much better between us?" Others know that there is more healing to be done, but fear "rocking the boat" or "stirring things up again" by focusing intensely on their coupleship.

If you relate to this, we encourage you to remember that any progress you made in your relationship so far has been the result of facing your individual and couples challenges head-on. It has been a long journey to this point, and no one would blame you if you stopped now. But because of your courage and effort, you have given yourselves an opportunity to do things within your relationship that were not possible before. The initial gains that have likely brought some relief to both of you have opened the door to the possibility of more significant change and wholesale shifts in your coupleship.

Think of the house of your dreams. Imagine that after much sacrifice to save for its expense, the plans have been drawn, the lot has been bought, and all the necessary materials and laborers are on the site. They are waiting for you to give them the green light to start construction, but you have some internal hesitation: "What if I'm unable to maintain it properly? What if something terrible happens and I'm unable to make the payments? What if I grow tired of the location? I could probably be fine staying in the home I have now, and not have to worry about all these things." You are in a similar position right now with your relationship: There is nothing that says you *must* realize your dreams, even when they are within your reach. On the other hand, there *is* a way of intimate relating that is now within your reach. We hope you agree that the effort and sacrifice required to get there will be rewarded in much the same way as your ongoing efforts and sacrifices in recovery have been rewarded so far.

2. Intensity vs. Intimacy:

One of the tensions often present in relationships is between intensity and intimacy. Intensity is often *mistaken* for intimacy. A couple can create a very intense, sexually stimulating situation with powerful orgasms by increasing risk, watching porn together, or even exchanging pain. Thus, they can experience high levels of arousal while being as *physically* close as two human beings can get, yet still be alone in their experiences. On the other hand, some couples that experience sexual boredom believe that the solution must involve turning up the intensity. Sometimes this couple will find something that does the trick (porn is a good example) but also finds that the effects are short-lived or that more external stimuli are needed to get the same effect or that one spouse becomes uncomfortable with new sexual activities that are pushing them beyond their personal boundaries. Despair usually follows.

Pursuing intensity chases intimacy away. Availing yourselves to intimacy allows you to let go and give yourselves to each other in a very passionate way. Yet, as this is occurring, it is essential that each spouse respect the other's comfort level. Sometimes there is an obvious difference in sexual comfort regarding any given sexual activity. The best way to handle this in the moment is to defer to the person who is least comfortable.

Some situations may benefit from negotiation if the person who is least comfortable thinks that the suggested sexual activity might not be off-limits, but would require some additional accommodations or conditions. For example, a husband may desire to give oral sex to his wife. She might realize that she is not comfortable with this, but might be willing to try it briefly if the lights are dim and if he promises to go as slowly and gently as she needs. In turn, her husband might understand that her discomfort has nothing to do with him, that it is merely her personal preference. He might also appreciate that his wife is allowing herself to consider *his* request and thereby making herself vulnerable. He has a chance to express his appreciation for her hearing his request and has an opportunity to respect her boundaries and thereby reinforce her trust in him. It is this trust that allows intimacy to deepen and allows their shared sexuality to continue to evolve.

Keeping the distinction between intimacy and intensity clear as you go through the SRT program will help you experience greater degrees of presence with each other. If you are accustomed to high-intensity sex, you may notice a feeling that "something is missing." This is normal and expected, and clears the way for the intimacy-based sexual relationship that will serve you well in an ongoing and renewable way.

3. Cybersex

When part of the sexual acting out behavior involves Cybersex or Internet pornography, we must confront the reality that many if not most recovering addicts miss the sexual intensity that only Cybersex can provide. The spouse of the Cybersex addict often struggles with feeling inadequate and wondering, "How am I supposed to compete with what you've been doing?" or "How can I compare with what you've been looking at?" It really is no competition. With its limitless menu, on-call availability and rapid-fire potential, the Internet has a capacity to stimulate the human brain that no spouse or partner can approach.

We must keep in mind that the pleasure centers of the brain (prominently the *nucleus accumbens*) were among the first areas of the brain to develop. Remarkably, in a span of just over a decade, the growth of Internet pornography and Cybersex has managed to stimulate the human brain *beyond its original design to process stimulation.* The cascade of dopamine that floods the pleasure centers while engaging in Cybersex leaves them craving more and more dopamine to get the same effect. That is why Cybersex has been referred to as the "crack cocaine" of sexual addiction. The good news is that even if you have been highly addicted to Internet porn and Cybersex, your brain is capable of changing through the process of recovery. It is entirely possible to choose to leave Cybersex behind, thereby trading false intimacy with images, fantasies or secret relationships, for *real intimacy* in your primary relationship.

4. Help! We're stuck in the past!

When a spouse or partner of a sex addict learns about the addict's secret life, it is like a bomb exploding: Pain, confusion, sorrow, anger, fear and even shame are the emotional shock waves that reverberate repeatedly, unexpectedly and undesirably. The spouse has suffered a real trauma, and needs to be treated as such. Beyond supporting the spouse with treatment that integrates PostTraumatic Stress Disorder (PTSD) and recovery principles, part of honoring the trauma involves the addict preparing a formal disclosure as well as an emotional restitution. It also involves the addict demonstrating a steady and consistent commitment to restoring trust through keeping one's word and actively embracing recovery.

However, sometimes after many months or years of the addict doing what s/he was "supposed" to do in recovery, the spouse or partner remains haunted by the painful past. Even when the couple has been doing well in recovery for a year or more, s/he might replay certain hurtful events over and over again in his/her mind, and might experience intense negative emotion around them. S/he may be triggered to become angry, withdrawn, critical or controlling. These ruminations, emotions and behaviors are often viewed in an over-simplified manner as a sign that the spouse is just "stuck." However, it often indicates that the spouse needs something more in order to move forward in his/her healing.

Using the process described in Chapter 4, *Revisiting Critical Incidents of Betrayal,* can be quite effective in these instances. The mutual benefit of this process is significant: The spouse can access the unresolved trauma that has been lurking beneath the surface, and can honor his/her feelings by sharing whatever they may be. The addict can reconnect with the healthy shame that *should* be there. Both participants are likely to feel a sense of release and a greater bond after being vulnerable through this experience together. Previously intrusive thoughts often become less frequent and less intense.

There are instances, however, when a spouse has extreme difficulty emerging from the acute pain surrounding those early weeks and months. Some simply want their spouse, who has caused so much pain, *fixed* once and for all. Many other spouses suffer in silence, paralyzed by the terrible pain and a non-existent list of attractive options. The common thread in these situations is that the spouse struggles to develop a recovery program of his/her own.

Andrea and Matt are a good example of this challenging profile. It started when Andrea noticed racy text messages on Matt's phone. When confronted, Matt denied anything inappropriate at first, but confessed his "Craigslist" habit the next day. It turned out that for 6 years he had been engaging in sexual relationships with women he met online. Matt promised to stop and sought treatment. Andrea threatened many times to leave Matt, and even consulted with a divorce attorney. Matt told Andrea that while he certainly hoped she would stay with him, that he understood how damaging his behaviors had been. He told her that his therapist suggested they prepare for a formal disclosure. Andrea wanted no part of "hearing all that awful stuff again." With the help of his therapist, Matt also prepared a clarification letter as part of an Emotional Restitution process, but Andrea wouldn't agree to participate in that process or even read the statement he had written. Matt expressed concern that he could see how much she was hurting, yet did not see her getting any support of her own. After nine months of his own treatment and eight months of sobriety, Matt bought her a book written for spouses and partners of sex addicts. It was as if another bomb went off.

Andrea said,

> "OK, so you go out and screw all these women behind my back, giving them gifts, spending OUR money on whores, exposing me to god knows what diseases and now I'm supposed to read a book to tell me that I had something to do with it? That I need to be in my *own* recovery? *You* were the one doing those awful things, *I* was the one living by our marriage vows and taking care of our kids and our home. Everyone says I should just be done with you, but if you want a chance at saving this relationship then stop telling me what I need to do- it's enough for me just to try to stop crying- you need to figure out why you're such an asshole! So when you and the good doctor have that part figured out, give me a call."

No one would or should argue that what happened in the relationship was "fair" to Andrea, and it is perfectly normal for her to feel the anger that she is feeling. However, if she cannot eventually find a way around the resentment she feels for Matt, their couple's recovery will be next to impossible. Without a recovery of her *own*, the best that their relationship can hope for is that they will stay married only on paper.

However, if she is able to honor the trauma she has been through by accepting support from others who know what her pain feels like, she might find herself more able to deal directly with the damage Matt has done. Eventually, she might be able to join Matt in taking responsibility for her side of the street while he is taking responsibility for his side. If so, then the upside potential for their relationship's deep healing and reconstruction increases dramatically. She might also find the courage to leave the relationship, if that is what she ultimately decides would be in her best interest. It is ironic that Andrea, like all spouses in her situation, did not ask for *any* of this pain, but holds so much influence regarding what comes of it.[11]

5. Cross-Addiction and Co-Morbidity

Sometimes one or both partners have other compulsive behaviors, such as drinking, gambling, over eating, that become more active when the sexually addictive behaviors are under control. Either spouse might have Attention Deficit Disorder or struggle with depression or anxiety, or with compulsive spending or eating. We need to be aware that if other addictions or mental health issues are not being treated, the risk of unintentionally sabotaging the SRT program increases. We believe that any delay in starting the SRT process that results from treating other such conditions is time well spent and ultimately will make the SRT process much more efficient.

6. Pre-existing sexual dysfunction or sexual dissatisfaction

It is very common for couples who have addiction in their relationship to also experience some sexual dysfunction such as low desire, difficulty with sexual arousal (e.g. erectile dysfunction or not feeling aroused), or difficulty with sexual release (difficulty reaching orgasm or controlling orgasm). Couples are challenged in two ways:

   a) *Couples need a way of understanding the dysfunction.* When recovering couples have experienced sexual dysfunction in their relationship, the couple often develops a narrative along the lines of, "None of this addictive stuff would have happened if our sex life was better to begin with." While it is a commonly held belief, it is too reductionistic, blaming and misleading. It is always helpful to get beyond some of the superficial explanations available: "Our sex life was too boring; it was always more important to him than to me; she was just too uptight about sex; he was never interested in my pleasure." While there may be some legitimacy to these and other complaints, there is always much more to be understood regarding how each spouse experienced their own sexual reality. Significant paradigm shifts need to be made regarding how you think about yourself as a sexual being and how you think about your shared sexual intimacy.

   b) *Couples need a specific treatment plan to address sexual problems.* It's not enough to trust that specific sexual problems will resolve themselves as a function of each partner working their respective recovery programs. However, the work of individual recovery most definitely *will* help each partner be in a better position to engage a process of sex therapy indicated for any given sexual problem. There are specific treatment protocols for sexual dysfunction and a variety of approaches available to address varying degrees and sources of sexual dissatisfaction. In the SRT program, a specific plan to intervene on any such

---

[11] For a more in-depth discussion of the co-addict's challenge, we recommend reading the "Should I Stay or Should I Go" chapter by Dr. Patrick Carnes in *Mending a Shattered Heart*.

issues would be indicated in conjunction with the fourth phase of treatment (Enhancement).

7. Toxic Fumes:

Blame, sarcasm, verbal attacks, belittling remarks are toxic. When one or both spouses see the other as their biggest problem, toxicity is the consistent byproduct. The communication style often descends into "attack and defend," and is characterized by mutual resentment. Each person has an air-tight case in their own minds that they are in the right, which means their partner is in the wrong. As each feels unfairly treated, they give themselves permission to even the score by becoming passive-aggressive (e.g. avoidance) or by using belittling remarks, name-calling, threats, sarcasm, manipulation, lies and blame. This is what is referred to as, "attacking from the victim position." When we see evidence of this kind of toxicity, it usually indicates the need for more individual work because of the chronic resentment. Many times, the introduction of the Talking and Listening Boundaries is enough to help a couple minimize the intensity and frequency of this toxic cycle (Appendix A).

8. Recovery = Feeling More:

Recovery is all about slowing our minds down and focusing on what we are thinking and feeling *before* we decide what we will be doing. Thus, when couples approach SRT in recovery, each spouse is likely to be much more connected to their inner worlds than ever. On paper, this certainly looks like a good thing, and it is! But it also makes the presence of a functional boundary system more important than ever. Functional boundaries help each spouse be better able to understand what they are feeling emotionally and what they are seeing and hearing from their spouse. Otherwise, there is a real risk of having a lot of unfiltered feelings flying around!

9. Allergic reactions to structure:

Some people have an initial or even an ongoing resistance to the structure involved in SRT. For example, we have heard complaints that, "This feels artificial, contrived, mechanical," etc. We try to validate that this is a normal reaction and acknowledge that most people **do** feel the effects of deliberately following a clearly defined and structured format. In fact, the foreign feelings that often accompany the early stages of SRT represent tangible proof that the couple is following their commitment to do things differently.

However, there are times when the initial feelings of awkwardness persist and become a distraction. In these cases, it is important to try to understand where the resistance is coming from. For example, in relationships where sex has served as a primary source of validation or a regulating mechanism (e.g. intense sex after an intense argument), people tend to have a lot of anxiety about being told that access to their sexual security blanket is going to need to change. This understandably often manifests as resistance to the structure.

In this and other instances of resistance, it is helpful to acknowledge that the anxiety (the resistance) is *an artifact of the addiction*. It is left over from the old ways of thinking about one's needs and wants and left over from the old fears about being in a relationship. Just as each spouse has been able to transcend their fears of change in early recovery, this is yet another opportunity to do so. We know of so many people who have come face to face with their resistance to structure who persevered and found a better way to be in sexual and intimate relationship with the one they love.

10. "For sex therapy, we are sure not having much sex!"

This is something we have heard in response to SRT's emphasis on slowing things down and enjoying sensual touch just for the sake of pleasure, and cultivating intimacy while learning how to be more relational. While there is a great deal of physical and emotional intimacy in the early stages of SRT, there is not much sexual touching. Thus, some participants are more aware of what they are missing than what they could be enjoying.

11. Biggest Needs, Biggest Problems

If you remember Angela and Dylan from the previous chapter, they fit a common pattern: Dylan's sexual *neediness* and his walled-off stance felt so big to Angela that it crowded out her *own* sexuality. Dylan's addictive thinking told him that sex is his biggest need and that sex is the highest form of love. In relationships, many sex addicts like Dylan initially look to their spouse as their "supplier," their main source of validation through the most powerfully validating experience they have ever had: Sex with another human being. When the rejection they experience becomes too painful, and resentment toward their spouse creeps in, many sex addicts like Dylan feel entitled to get this "biggest need" satisfied by any means necessary. Sometimes this means acting out sexually with people other than one's spouse or using pornography to intensify the fantasy about having sex with people other than one's spouse. It took some time, but Dylan was eventually able to understand that while he had done well to curtail his acting out behaviors, he also needed to examine how he went through many aspects of the classic addictive cycle in his shared sexuality with Angela.

For example, one of Dylan's previous patterns was to kiss and touch Angela just as she was about to fall asleep at night. She would usually give in to his advances. But if he tried to move things toward sexual activities with which she was uncomfortable, she would say something along the lines of, "Look, if you want to have sex, we'll have sex. But I'm too tired to try anything like that tonight." Dylan would typically accept the "vanilla sex," but felt rejected in the process. Feelings of resentment usually followed for both: Angela resented Dylan for continually not respecting her need for rest, and Dylan resented Angela for continually rejecting him.

The resentment provided the fuel for each to elevate the other to the lofty status of *"My Biggest Problem in the World."* It followed logically that they were also feeling so dependent on each other to *relieve* them of their biggest problem. This created a vicious cycle of focusing on each other's behaviors and making negative assumptions about those behaviors. These assumptions were consistent with each one's core beliefs around not being loveable, not being able to depend on others, not mattering, etc.

Variations of this distance creating dance are as frequent as a common cold in relationships. However, when addiction is present, it is more like pneumonia, because of the dysfunctional and destructive ways in which addicts and spouses think about themselves and react to each other.

In a completely different situation, some spouses are shocked to learn of the addict's secret life, not because s/he has been good at concealing behavior, but because the addict had shown *so little interest* in sex in their marriage. The shock often turns quickly to anger, especially if the spouse has been dissatisfied with their sexual frequency. The addict's lack of sexual interest in the primary relationship is usually either an avoidance strategy regarding intimacy (commonly a passive way of acting out feelings of resentment toward the spouse) or a function of the addict's ever-increasing need for stimulation and intensity that has made sexual intimacy with a spouse less preferred to high risk/high intensity sexual acting out experiences.

Conclusion:

Each of these eleven barriers will hold the most power over you when it is not acknowledged. With that in mind, take a moment to review where you might foresee issues with one or more of the above barriers. For now, just consider what barriers *you* might have. Trust that as long as you are willing to be real about any barrier being there, the way around your barriers will become clearer.

7

SRT Goals and Components

Goals:

Now that you are ready to begin Sexual Reintegration Therapy, you need to have a solid grasp of the specific therapeutic goals around which the program is centered. The following are the key design concepts that underlie the SRT Program. Each one represents an action step that you will take as part of your SRT experience. (You might notice that some of these are already areas of competence or even strengths for you). SRT has been designed to:

1. **Identify unhealthy patterns of intimacy blocks and allow you to work toward transcending them.**

   Living in fear of one's spouse is a terrible way to go through life. However, this is the root of all intimacy disorders: a fundamental fear of relating with another in a deep and meaningful way. *In the SRT model, a system of healthy, intimate relating is established as the new normal.* Gradually, you will be able to share more authentically with each other. You will be able to identify when you need assistance and will ask for it in an appropriate way. You will be able to respect and accept that your spouse will not always be able to meet your needs, even when you make yourself vulnerable and summon up the courage to ask for something that is important to you. You will be less threatened when your spouse has a different thought or feeling than you do. Trust increases as you observe each other actively pursuing significant change in your lives.

2. **Facilitate a searching and honest self-assessment of each of your contributions to the dysfunction in your relationship.**

   You may have heard the old adage, "A system is only as strong as its weakest link." Applied to recovering marriages, the "weak link" manifests in the form of resistance to looking inward at how one has unintentionally contributed to the problems in the relationship. The extent to which you can take responsibility for keeping your own side of the street clean (and avoid the cycle of blaming each other) is the extent to which you will be able to heal your wounded coupleship and give it new life. A commitment to full ownership of personal responsibility removes any "ceiling" on your potential for a full and deep healing process. The SRT program guides you in looking inward, seeing what is there, and sharing what you find with each other.

61

3. **Facilitate a deep personal reflection on your sexual selves, and how your sexual self has interacted with your spouse's sexual self.**

It never occurs to most to focus thought on how we have evolved into the sexual beings we are. Usually, this type of thinking is only prompted when there is an obvious sexual problem. If you are reading this book, your situation likely qualifies as one of those "obvious problems." One great irony is that in many cases we would never have attained the depth of knowledge, growth or healing that we have achieved were it not for the pain that was thrust upon us. While no one would intentionally set out to suffer from such emotional pain, since you have found it, (or it found you) now you are confronted with choosing how to deal with it. In order to deal with it, you must understand it.

That is where reflecting on how your sexual self developed and understanding how that sexual self has interacted with your spouse's sexual self comes in. The first step involves understanding yourself. SRT will help you take a thorough inventory of the messages you received about your sexuality as child and how those messages shaped the ways you think and feel about sex and how you behave sexually. Similarly, SRT will help you reflect on earlier sexual experiences to assess how they have been influential in your sexual evolution.

When you and your spouse have finished your self-assessments, the second step involves looking at what happens when these two sexual selves interact with each other. You will learn to recognize how the patterns you identify in your sex life (who initiates, how often; who leads, who follows; how each of you feels before and after sex; comfort with touch, spontaneity, experimentation, etc.) are functions of the evolutions of these two sexual selves. These selves evolved largely before the two of you ever met. Often the process of looking at your sex life from this detached, observational perspective helps to lessen feelings of blame and resentment that may be present.

4. **Facilitate a safe framework to share your growing awareness.**

It is one thing for you to be developing increasing levels of awareness and understanding regarding your individual and shared sexuality on your own. It is quite another to share this unfolding awareness in an appropriately authentic way with your spouse. To experience some anxiety around the prospect of allowing your true self, including your feelings, values, boundaries, needs, wants and preferences, to be known by another is quite common. It is common to experience even *more* anxiety around the prospect of revealing such things when the subject is sex. Even the most severe sex addicts, with all their sexual experiences, often struggle to communicate sexually in an effective or appropriate manner with their spouse. So we know that the *amount* of sexual activity someone has had does not necessarily make them skilled in dialoguing about it. Pioneering sexuality researchers Masters and Johnson long ago proclaimed the critical importance of being able to communicate openly about sexuality in intimate relationships. In fact, they could not have been clearer in attributing this skill as a basic, foundational element for healthy and mutually satisfying sex lives.

By working the SRT program, you will be guided in developing greater skill and comfort in talking about your sexuality. You will learn a framework for sharing your sexual realities with each other based on Pia Mellody's model of "Functional Boundaries."[14] It is designed to keep these conversations safe and manageable so that you may experience more comfort and less anxiety while discussing your sexual realities authentically. As you gradually experience being able to share your sexual wants, needs, preferences, feelings and boundaries and feel more safety while doing it, you will be able to achieve a depth of intimacy that would not otherwise be possible. It is in this way that you will experience a paradigm shift: That which was unknowable and unmentionable is now known and shared. *This is consistent with living in abundance, as you are not limited by the fear of reality or by the fear of how your spouse might respond to knowing your reality.* You trust your ability to decide what to share, and to set boundaries with your spouse as needed.

5. **Facilitate a shared vision of your healthy sexual selves becoming an integrated whole in your recovering marriage.**

We are learning more and more about the brain's *neuroplasticity* (its ability to grow new neuronal networks when it experiences certain processes of change).[15] One of those is the process of visualization. Just as many world class athletes have discovered and utilized the technique of visualizing success as a key component of their actual success, so too can recovering couples. SRT will help you to create a vision of your new life together, both inside and outside the bedroom. So much of early recovery is necessarily focused on saying "no" to destructive and unhealthy behaviors. Yet, being oriented to avoiding "off-limits" behavior will only take you so far.

Now it is time to turn your attention to what you can confidently and enthusiastically say "YES" to. The process of carefully creating a vision for how you would like to be in relationship with your spouse is empowering because *you* are the one doing the creating. Nothing is being put upon you, and you are not naively falling into patterns or situations. You both are beyond that by now. Your eyes are wide open to your own dysfunctional tendencies as well as how you have experienced dysfunction in relationship with your spouse. When you are firmly in touch with how you have been dysfunctional, the functional path becomes clearer. By working the SRT program, you will be able to clearly visualize this path and develop strategies to take you ever closer to that vision.

6. **Provide a structured approach necessary to help you achieve that vision.**

Often couples generally agree about what has been dysfunctional, and what would be more functional, but *still* experience frustration with their inability to make significant change in the relationship. What is often missing is a focused and consistent strategy and a clearly structured approach.

Structure is helpful in several ways. It helps to keeps things predictable, which translates into greater feelings of safety. Many recovering spouses grew up in family systems characterized by *un*predictability (e.g. unpredictable anger, unpredictable emotional attunement and/or meeting of basic needs, etc.) which placed them at risk for developing intimacy blocks later in their adult relationships.

Structure also promotes a legitimate basis for hope. For example, if you knew of two people, and each had a goal to lose 20 pounds, would you be more optimistic for success about the one that was following an established weight loss program or about the one doing it on his own? Odds are you would say the one who is following a program would have a better chance to reach the goal. Similarly, when you jointly commit as a couple to a clearly defined, structured program of change, like SRT, you can be confident that it has been successful for many others and that you are not on your own anymore. Furthermore, you can trust that if you stumble, you will have a safety net in place: The structure of a program that can accommodate challenges and can hold the path steady, regardless of any obstacles along the way.

7. **Provide new ways to embrace the anxieties and uncertainties that often exist in intimate romantic relationships as tolerable, manageable and informative.**

To be in a relationship with another person means that you will be out of sync with that person at least from time to time. There is no way around this fundamental truth because as two separate individuals, you are bound to have competing needs with each other, values that differ, opinions that are at odds, and different ideas about how to handle life's challenges. This is *normal and expected*. What becomes *problematic* is when couples develop a pattern of avoidance strategies to cope with many of these situations.

There are a wide range of possible triggers for one or both spouses to feel threatened by their perceived inability to negotiate a successful outcome. When someone experiences a negative emotion; when a spouse hears a complaint or criticism; when a spouse experiences anger toward or from their mate; when one spouse asks for help or is asked for help; when a spouse is not available to the other; when a spouse feels like s/he has been victimized by the other; when a spouse experiences sexual desire or becomes aware of the other's sexual desire. Perhaps you can think of situational triggers for your own avoidant response.

It sometimes can be difficult to identify actual avoidance strategies. For example, it's easy to see how leaving the house in anger, slamming a door, name-calling, and overworking can be avoidance strategies. But what about over-pursuing your spouse sexually? Or assuming a victim stance by keeping yourself quiet and withdrawn because of how wronged you believe you have been? How about buying an expensive piece of jewelry or even just flowers to smooth things over? What about accepting them? All of these behaviors and attitudes serve the same function: They prevent spouses from communicating about their real needs, their legitimate hurts, and their genuine fears. They all work against authentic intimacy.

64

We are likely to employ these types of strategies whenever we experience a threat. The threats can be highly subjective, completely internal and within us. Experiencing a personal need or even a personal preference can trigger this type of threat response. It can happen so quickly, that we are unaware of it happening!

How could a basic need or preference create such an internal stir? In a word, the answer is "history." Long before you ever knew each other, you received intense training around how others heard and responded to your needs. This training is commonly referred to as "childhood." So did you learn that the people you were supposed to be able to trust were trustworthy? Did you learn that the people who were supposed to be there for you showed up consistently? Did you learn that your worth was a constant or did it vary because you had to earn it by performing, excelling, caretaking, or entertaining?

Whatever you learned originally, you were likely to have those lessons reinforced in the adult relationships you formed. One common result: Instead of finding an appropriate way to share authentically what we really think, feel, want or need, we withdraw, pacify, criticize, become sexual (or asexual) or we assume a victim stance. It can feel like the relationship must be abnormal because it is so difficult.

SRT will help you learn to tolerate the normal and expected tensions around natural areas of conflict in your coupleship. You will learn that the greatest gift you can exchange with each other is the gift of your *authenticity* - how you really *feel*, what you really *desire*, who you really *are*. You will learn that when you do experience needs or wants that are in conflict with each other, you will be able to respectfully negotiate a successful outcome.

The result of any successful negotiation (whether in the boardroom or the bedroom) is that both sides come away from the negotiation feeling that they are "OK." As you get more experience with successful negotiation around your needs and wants, you *will not need* the avoidance strategies that you once used to protect yourself from the inevitable disappointment or frustration you learned to expect. In this way, you may achieve another paradigm shift: "When I experience a need, want or preference, or have a thought or opinion, *I can move toward my spouse with authenticity instead of hiding my authentic self behind my fears.*" This is the essence of intimacy.

Relationships *are* inherently challenging, and it would be much simpler to go it alone. But accepting the expected challenges and practicing respectful, direct communication allows us to enjoy the limitless benefits of being in relationship while keeping the truly difficult moments to a minimum.

8. **Provide planned opportunities to connect with each other in more relaxed and enjoyable ways inside and outside of the bedroom.**

Part of the structure of SRT involves spouses scheduling time with each other. We call these times "Planned Intimate Experiences," or "PIEs." More than anything, the couples' ability to schedule their time with each other and honor their commitments to those times, is important for success in the SRT program. This makes sense because in order for any good to come from a program that involves two people working closely together, both people must *show up* at the same place and the same time and be prepared to join together on whatever is planned. Because this is so fundamental, we do not leave it to chance. We strongly encourage you to be good schedulers with each other, planning the dates and times for your PIEs just as you would plan a meeting with your boss at work, or with your child's teacher.

This is typically a new way of doing things. For most of us, our couple time is the first thing to be displaced when life's demands are calling and our time becomes more constricted. For this reason, most couples experience some initial tension to find time for their PIEs. We have yet to find a couple who has thought, "I was hoping someone would tell me what to do with all the free time I have on my hands these days! Fantastic!" The reality is that we are busier and more "plugged in" than ever, placing a real premium on our time.

However, when you find a way to make time for each other, you are sending a loud and clear message: *"I value you and our relationship enough to carve out this time in our busy lives."* If you are like so many of our couples, you might feel momentum building as you become consistent in scheduling time together and honoring the commitment to that time. In this way, you may achieve another paradigm shift: When at one time you may have felt helpless, hopeless and stuck as a couple, you now see and believe that *you can work together in partnership.*

9. Address specific sexual problems and dissatisfaction

Many couples seek therapy because of specific sources of sexual dissatisfaction or diagnosable sexual disorders. Examples include: Low desire (male and female); erectile dysfunction; low arousal (female); premature ejaculation; inhibited orgasmic disorder (male and female); and painful intercourse. Couples in recovery from sex addiction seem to experience higher frequencies of sexual dissatisfaction and dysfunction than the general population. The reasons are numerous, but perhaps the best place to look is Dr. Patrick Carnes' Core Belief #4: "Sex is my greatest need." This changes everything as far as sexual satisfaction is concerned. Why? Because we know that *sex works best and is the most satisfying when it is free of any demands, pressures, or performance expectations.* When sex is elevated to the top or near the top of one's hierarchy of needs, it takes on more than it can be expected to handle. Consequently, we start to see the types of complaints and disorders mentioned previously.

One of the goals of SRT is to *put sex back in its place.* When sex finds its way back to its appropriate place in your life, a tremendous weight is lifted from your shared sexual intimacy. You are then in a much better position to enjoy each other as you are free from this pressure. This is tricky because some recovering addicts and their spouses experience huge swings in their sexual feelings as they move through various stages of recovery. If you can relate to this dizzying roller coaster, there are many ways to understand them, depending on your specific circumstances. Some addicts and spouses shut down sexually in early recovery. Others report a marked increase in frequency of sexual activity in their recovering relationships. Whatever it has been for you, the likelihood is that you have been making it up as you go along. There is no denying the fact that we are all sexual beings. SRT provides you with a proven model for deciding proactively *how* you would like to be as sexual beings, and as sexual beings in relationship with each other.

The paradigm shift from being sexually reactive to sexually proactive can be incredibly empowering for both of you. It is much like the creation of a "Healthy Sex Plan" that many recovering addicts complete as part of their Relapse Prevention Plan. In SRT, you will connect with specific, healthy sexual attitudes and behaviors. You will have a chance to claim them, internalize them and to develop a lifestyle that supports them. The likelihood of having a consistently satisfying, deepening sexual connection increases accordingly.

10. **Create a clearly defined plan for enjoying sexual and emotional intimacy that is based upon all of the gains you made during the SRT program.**
    The SRT program's finish line is reached when you create your *"Lifetime Blueprint for Functional Sexual Intimacy and Abundance."* This is a concrete document you will create that highlights the many gains you will have made. You will address how to maintain each of these gains as part of the Blueprint in order to promote an ongoing practice of what you now know to be keys to your success (please also refer to the description of the Lifetime Blueprint in the "Components" section below).

Components:
The process of working through the SRT program can take several formats. Some couples may wish to attempt to take themselves through the program simply by using this book. While this may be possible for some, *we strongly recommend having a Certified Sex Addiction Therapist (CSAT) to guide you through this program.* This way, you can have the benefit of that professional's understanding of the specific nature of the challenges you are undertaking. Each spouse is likely to encounter some fears, insecurities and uncertainty as part of the process, and it is very helpful to be able to process those feelings with a guide so they may be properly understood and honored.

There are several components to the process of working the SRT Program:
1. **Five-Phase model:** The program is divided into five distinct phases, each with its own specific focus. Each phase utilizes a combination of highly structured experiences to achieve specific goals.
2. **Mutual Agreements:** At the beginning of each phase, you are asked to read a series of statements aloud and discuss them. Each spouse is then asked to initial each statement to formally indicate your agreement with the statement. This is both a practical and symbolic way of helping you to enter each new phase feeling unified in agreement along some very meaningful dimensions. If either of you is unclear regarding the meaning of the statement, there is an opportunity

to discuss it together. Likewise, if either of you is uncomfortable with some aspect of the statement, you are encouraged to discuss whatever the issue or concern might be.

3. **Planned Intimate Experiences (PIE):** After completing the Mutual Agreements for any given phase, you are ready to engage the Planned Intimate Experiences contained in each phase.

   The key word is "planned." One of the first challenges you will encounter is *creating the time* that is necessary for the experience to occur. SRT works best when you dedicate approximately three PIE times every week with each other.

   When time is tight, couple time is usually the first thing to go. If you have a standing "Date Night" with each other, how many times have you moved or canceled it over the past several months? Most people would answer with a number greater than zero. An endless number of things can "bump" couple time: Working late, the kids' homework, phone calls, requests from family or friends, the TV show you just can't miss, the errand or email that just can't wait until tomorrow. Granted, some things simply cannot be helped such as when a child is sick, or if you must occasionally work late. While there may be legitimate reasons for postponing your dedicated couple time, our hope is that you jointly and deliberately raise the threshold for those postponements, thereby giving your couple time a higher level of priority. We have found that, *the variable that is most highly correlated with couples' success in the SRT program is the ability to schedule PIE times with each other and to consistently honor those commitments.*

When you get together for your PIE times, the PIEs will fall under three categories.[16]

   a. **Communication Experiences:** The Communication Experiences involve responding to written worksheet questions on specific topics that are completed by each of you on your own time, and then shared during your scheduled PIE time. They have two primary purposes. First, they help each of you to know yourselves better through the reflective nature of the exercise. Second, they help you become more skilled and comfortable in sharing back and forth what you know and what you are learning about yourselves.
   b. **Sensual Experiences:** These are the PIEs that involve touching each other in ways that are clearly defined in the instructions that precede each experience. Each sensual experience has a communication element to it, as you will be asked to make notes about what you just experienced and to discuss with each other.
   c. **Educational Experiences:** Several of the experiences have an educational component. It may involve learning about your body, your

spouse's body, male and female sexual response, or learning about how to most effectively and safely communicate with each other.

4. Lifetime Blueprint for Functional Sexual Intimacy and Abundance:

At the conclusion of the SRT Program, you will be asked to create an action plan that is based on all you have learned through the program. This document is called the *"Lifetime Blueprint for Functional Sexual Intimacy and Abundance."* We recommend that you to refer to this document consistently after completing this program and to ask yourselves, "How are we doing?" It allows you to maintain the progress and growth for which they worked so hard and to do so in a way that is efficient and manageable.

***

Now that you are familiar with the design concepts behind SRT and the various components of the program, you are ready to read in Chapter 8 about the specific guidelines for working your way through the PIEs.

8

SRT Playbook

Getting Started:

Once you have agreed on a date and time for any given PIE, record it in Appendix C. You will also notice that there is space provided to record whose turn it is to be the "initiator." The initiator is the person who is basically responsible for calling your PIE time to order. For the caressing PIEs, it is also the initiator's job to set up the room in a way that feels *honoring of the experience to follow*. That phrase will appear repeatedly in the instructions for the caressing PIEs. It is intentionally vague because it can take many different forms. It might mean simply tidying up, or it could mean adjusting the lighting, putting on music, having extra pillows or blankets accessible, etc. Here is a practical example of what it might look like to be the initiator: Let's say your next scheduled PIE was for 8:30 PM on Wednesday. As the initiator, it is your job to find your spouse at 8:30PM on Wednesday and simply let him/her know a) that you are ready, and b) where you'll be waiting. If it was to be a caressing PIE, you would have already prepared the room in advance of your start time. The structure of this system is designed to take any uncertainty and guesswork out of the process of getting started.

When you have both arrived, *the first thing you will do is to read aloud the "Purpose and Goals" and "Instructions" that introduce each PIE.* You might notice that some phrases repeat themselves from one PIE to the next. This is done intentionally to reinforce design concepts that are important to practice consistently throughout the entire program. Finally, it will be very important for each of you to *have a journal or notebook in which you can record the thoughts and feelings you have in response to the PIEs.*

Caressing PIEs

The caressing experiences are designed to build gradually upon each other. During these experiences, you will take turns in the acts of giving and receiving pleasure through sensual touch. The touch to be used is different than the deep type of touch that is great for massaging a sore or tight muscle group. Instead, the type of touch being used in the SRT program is a *light, skin to skin caress*. This type of touch is an excellent way that you can communicate your care, trust and nurturance for each other.

A visualization that can be helpful is to imagine all of the caresser's feelings of affection, care and love flowing freely from his/her fingertips into the body of the receiver. There is no right or wrong way to caress or to receive a caress. This is designed to be an interactive experience that is *structured but not scripted*: There are an endless number of possible experiences within the structure. Some people worry that the structure of scheduling and following instructions will eliminate any spontaneity. On the contrary, there is plenty of room for spontaneity within the structure as each spouse is encouraged to be mindful of anything that would make their own experience more comfortable, pleasurable and fun.

While progressing through the SRT program, it is very important not to go beyond the level of physical intimacy relative to where you are currently in the program. For example, it is not recommended to have intercourse until it is arrived at within the structure of the program. For some, this may amount to a celibacy period, and people have experienced this with varying degrees of discomfort. In essence, you are engaging in a purification process for your sexual intimacy which consists of the following principles:

- When addiction is present, any sexual activity that has been occurring between you has necessarily been affected by the addiction and co-addiction. (e.g. sex as validating your worth; sex as way to manage negative feeling states; sex as way to control another's sexual sobriety, sex as a sign that "We're OK.").
- You are now in the process of creating a new, healthier version of your sexual intimacy. Therefore, it becomes important to stop doing things the "old way" as you are trying to create something new.
- There is a need to slow things down in order to be fully present and available to engage in the process of giving and receiving pleasure just for the pleasure itself, not for any end goal or expectation.
- The idea is that when you reach the part of the SRT program that involves intercourse, it will be a different experience than before. This is because you will have learned to be more present with each other, to appreciate pleasurable touch without any demands or expectations for arousal or performance and to claim a sexual intimacy that neither of you could have known without each other.

Now we will review in detail each of the two roles that you will play during the caressing PIEs.[17]

Receiver:

As the receiver, your main responsibility is to be as present as possible with yourself and your spouse so you can soak up as much pleasure as possible. The basic idea is that as the receiver, *you are responsible for your own pleasure*. As the owner of your pleasure, you will need to *have an idea* about what would feel most comfortable, pleasurable or fun, and also to be able to *express* it appropriately. This involves a significant paradigm shift for many people who may have naturally assumed that their spouse was responsible for the quality of any given experience of physical or sexual intimacy. The most common sexual fantasy just might be, "Well s/he should *know* what I like!"

71

The term used for asking for what you would like while being caressed (so the above fantasy is more likely to become a reality) is "redirection." It is not simply telling someone *what* to do, but asking your spouse to modify what s/he is doing. Sometimes an effective redirection takes the form of teaching ("I'm really enjoying this, but could you please try using a circular touch like this?"). It is natural to experience some vulnerability when re-directing. This is because you are allowing yourself to be known ("This is what feels good/might feel good") and asking someone to help you. As such, there is a great deal of mutual trust involved. The receiver trusts that the caresser will hear the redirection non-defensively, and the caresser trusts that the receiver *will* redirect whenever necessary. This is a much different process than what is often the case, such as hoping your spouse will catch on to your non-verbal cues or resenting that your spouse isn't more "adventurous."

It is essential that as the receiver you not only ask directly for what you would like, but also have respect for the caresser's response. For example, the receiver might ask his wife if she could spend more time caressing his genitals, but she might be uncomfortable with his request and would need to communicate her reality to him.

The receiver always needs to know that s/he can stop the caressing if it becomes too uncomfortable at any time and for any reason. Sometimes, this might involve asking to take a break or to switch roles (e.g. "I'm feeling a little anxious right now, so I think I'd like to just have you hold me without any caressing and see how that feels;" e.g. "What you're doing has felt so nice, but I can tell that I'm getting nervous again, would you be open to me caressing you for a while to see how it goes?"). While often difficult, moments like these can be opportunities to enhance trust, acceptance and empathy.

Finally, it is often the case that the receiver becomes so relaxed by some forms of sensual touch that s/he may tend toward drifting off to sleep. While relaxation is a wonderful benefit of the sensual experience, it is necessary to stay awake in order to be present for the experience of shared intimacy. If you find yourself struggling to stay awake or notice that your spouse is drifting off, pause and consider if it is a good idea to switch roles, vary the experience, or in some cases even to postpone the experience.

Caresser:

As the caresser, you will have the opportunity and privilege of enjoying your spouse's body in a very sensual way. You will be using a light, skin to skin type of touch on specific areas of your spouse's body as directed in the instructions for each caressing PIE. It is very important that the caresser honor and respect the boundaries of the instructions, as this can be a helpful component of building trust.

Sometimes as the caresser you may feel uncertain regarding how to touch in a way that feels pleasurable to your spouse. The best strategy is to *let your enjoyment of your spouse's body guide your caressing.* This will allow you to be more presently connected with your own experience of the moment.

While following this principle, it is also important to trust that your spouse is enjoying the caressing unless s/he offers a redirection. In that case, you have an opportunity to appreciate the trust involved in making a redirection. You can choose a gracious, generous and grateful spirit as you open yourself to your spouse's request.

This often requires a shift in how you interpret your spouse's redirection: It is NOT a critique, but a fully functional and necessary request for something different. It certainly does not mean you are doing anything wrong.

You can monitor your *internal listening boundary* (Appendix A) in order to receive redirection in a functional manner. For example, upon hearing your wife's request that you try a circular motion while caressing her rather than a vertical motion, instead of thinking, "I can never do anything right with this woman," or "Why does she always have to tell me what I'm doing wrong?" your internal listening boundary would help you know that her request is about *her*, not about *you*. The part in this example that *is* about you is that she trusts you enough to offer the redirection in the first place. Being present enough to appreciate such vulnerable moments will help to sustain a well-founded hopefulness.

Before concluding the Playbook, we offer guidance around a common question: "How much time should we spend in each role (caresser/receiver)?" We emphasize NOT being so concerned about the length of time. Having exactly equal amounts of time in each role is not as important as being as present as you can with each moment of your PIE time together. The only caveat is that is does take *some* time to really connect, to achieve a desired state of presence. The balance lies in allowing yourself *enough* time to connect as fully as possible in each role without feeling any time *pressure*.

***

You are now ready to begin the SRT Program in Part Two of this book. As you do, know that the reading and preparation you have done to this point has positioned you to enjoy a rich, exciting and rewarding experience together.

PART II:
Working the
Sexual Reintegration Therapy Program

9
Phase I: Shared Commitment

As you stand poised to begin the SRT Program, it is likely that you both want the same things: To feel free to enjoy each other, to share life's pleasures together and to know sexual intimacy as you have never known it before. There is no stronger foundation for the healing you desire than knowing you are aligned on the same side of this journey. You have already faced fire all around, and you chose to stay and defend your home. By now, you are ready for it to not feel like such a struggle. You are ready to redeem the pain you have endured and to open yourselves to new ways of being in relationship with each other. The possibility of building a new future together, a future based in respect and integrity that will infuse all aspects of your intimacy is closer than ever before.

The first phase of Sexual Reintegration Therapy emphasizes this mutual investment that you both are making in your relationship. It begins with each of you formally choosing to engage in this shared process of healing, growth and discovery by completing and signing the SRT Commitment Contract. You are then directed to Appendix A where you will be introduced to the practice of Functional Boundaries. Also in this phase, each of you is asked to reflect on what you already have: The qualities you appreciate in each other that promote feelings of attraction. You will connect with your hopes and visions for your new relationship. You will be guided in establishing new ways of talking about things that matter to you. This type of deliberate and thoughtful sharing is a key component of intimacy, and as such carries with it some feelings of risk and vulnerability. You may be asked to share more than ever before, but you will not be asked to do so without some protection. The protection comes in the form of practicing a functional boundary system, which will be taught in this phase. Throughout this phase, you will be reminded to try to be empathic with your spouse, as s/he is likely finding this healing work as challenging as you are.

Before proceeding, please be sure that each of you has read the SRT Playbook so you are familiar with the guidelines and format of the program you are about to begin.

The SRT Commitment Contract is the first task you are asked to complete in this phase. It is a formal way for both of you to indicate that you willingly choose to invest and risk the emotional energy, vulnerability and commitment that will be involved in the SRT program. The contract includes a written acknowledgement of the <u>other's</u> greatest concerns about the process you are entering into and their needs (requests) that grow out of those concerns. Before signing the contract, you will need to ask each other what those concerns might be and also what might be helpful to your spouse.

75

SRT Commitment Contract
(Bercaw & Bercaw)

We understand that we are entering into an agreement to work together as partners toward the goal of creating a mutually satisfying relationship characterized by healthy emotional and sexual intimacy.

I understand that my spouse's greatest concern regarding this process is:

_____

_____

_____

(spouse initial _____)

Regarding the above concern, I understand that my spouse is requesting that I:

_____

_____

_____

(spouse initial _____)

I promise to continue to practice specific components of my recovery program while I am engaged in the SRT program including:

_____

_____

_____

By signing below, I pledge my commitment to work with my spouse in this process until it is complete and we both agree that we have created a healthy, new process of physical and emotional connecting that we can maintain.

_____   _____
Name   Date

Mutual Agreements: *Shared Commitment*

(Bercaw & Bercaw)

The Mutual Agreements reinforce the commitment you each make to each other and to this process. You are asked to read them aloud together and to initial in the space provided next to each one to indicate your agreement. (If you are not sure that you agree, please circle the statement and remember to discuss it with your spouse and therapist).

1. Our intimacy and sexuality deserve and need special healing. _____

2. We pledge our commitment to see this part of our healing through. _____

3. We will ask for support when we need it and will lend it when we are available. _____

4. We resolve to do the work required to transform what has been a weakness in our coupleship (intimacy) into a new strength. _____

5. We will use the same deliberate, competency-based approach that has taken us this far in recovery. _____

6. Our recovery journey is leading us into a life of abundance; let us allow our sexual selves to be part of this abundance. _____

Shared Commitment
Action Steps

- Agree to walk through this process together
- Connect with frustrations and fears as well as hopes and visions
- Learn Functional Boundaries
- Cultivate atmosphere of empathic support

Shared Commitment Planned Intimate Experience:

Practicing Functional Boundaries
(Bercaw & Bercaw)

Purpose and Goals:

You have by now read many references to boundaries in the earlier sections of this book. Practicing functional boundaries is foundational when trying to build a relationship that is grounded in respect and desirous of greater intimacy. Important as they are, boundaries are not part of our schooling or other training. As such, they need to be learned and practiced in adulthood.

Instructions:

Please turn to Appendix A in the back of the book for a detailed explanation of the model we want you to learn and practice. It is fine if you want to read this section on your own at some point, but be sure to read all parts of it aloud while you are together for this PIE.

Shared Commitment Planned Intimate Experience:

Attraction in Action
(Bercaw & Bercaw)

Purpose and Goals:
During the early stages of Sexual Reintegration Therapy, it is so important to cultivate awareness of the genuine, positive feelings you have for each other. It is equally important to be clear about how you might be able to feel even closer and *more* attracted to your spouse.

Instructions:
Each spouse is asked to make two lists:

1. Make a list that includes all of the characteristics your spouse possesses that make him/her attractive to you. These can be personality characteristics, physical characteristics or anything you can think of. What attracted you to your spouse in the first place? Also think about what you did not know about your spouse in the beginning of your relationship that you know now and find attractive (e.g. "What a great mother you are" "How you would overcome the adversity you have"). Do not worry about how long your list is, just focus on whatever is true for you.

2. The second list is to be limited to no more than two items. The title of the list is to be: "What would make my spouse even more attractive to me." (e.g. "If you would put your coffee mug in the dishwasher before leaving for work"; If you would look at me when we're talking so I know you're with me.") These items are negotiable and are not absolutes.

    Meet with your spouse to discuss your lists, starting with the first. After each of you has shared your lists, consider the following questions:
    *   Did you hear anything from your spouse that was a pleasant surprise?
    *   What did you find most meaningful in your spouse's list of your attractive qualities?
    *   Was there anything you had hoped to hear, but did not?

    Next, move to the second list, taking care to avoid critical and defensive statements. (The *Guidelines for Communicating* section in Appendix A may be helpful with sharing the second list.)

Shared Commitment Planned Intimate Experience:

Daily Shares
(Bercaw & Bercaw)

Purpose and Goals:

Nothing will promote intimacy more than consistently sharing your authentic selves with each other. To do this is to directly counter and reverse the avoidance strategies that you may be familiar with. While consistency is key, (as indicated by the "Daily" part of the title) this need not be an unnecessarily time-consuming process: Three to five minutes with Daily Shares can absolutely help you stay more connected. You will know at least a little more about each other and will be known a little bit more than before. Sometimes, you may find yourselves choosing to discuss in greater detail part of your Daily Shares. There is also something to be said for the process of "just showing up" as you keep this commitment to each other. Each time you follow through and make yourself available you send a message: "This time is important to me, and when I say I'm going to do something, I do." This helps in the restoration of trust and building of confidence in your relationship.

Instructions:

First, agree to meet at a specific time near the end of the day or evening. Eventually you may have a set time each evening for your Daily Shares, but in the beginning you might want to experiment and negotiate to see what works best. This process also can work fine over the phone if you cannot meet in person. After sitting down and becoming comfortable, you each will take a turn sharing with the other using the format below:

1. **Express an affirmation**. The only criterion for this affirmation is that it is a positive statement that is true for you. Examples:
   - "I appreciate your work ethic."
   - "I really admire the way you handled that situation even though it must not have been easy for you."
   - "I really felt close to you when you put your arm around me last night."
   - "I think you smell great!"

2. **Share something from your day.** It could be something that feels big, or perhaps something that feels light or even trivial.. Examples:
   - "I ran into Melissa when I was at lunch and I realized how much I miss her friendship."
   - "I tried calling the computer support line again but they made me wait forever and I had to hang up before I was even able to talk with anyone- so I was really frustrated and I'm starting to worry that it will never get fixed."
   - "I overheard Caleb explaining to Ashley that the tooth fairy will only leave money under the pillow if the tooth doesn't have any cavities. They are so funny sometimes!"

80

3. **Share something that's on your radar: A hope, dream, vision or concern.** It could be something way off on the horizon, or something that is with you right now. Examples:
   - "I'm really looking forward to our date on Friday."
   - "I'm starting to think more about changing my career path"
   - "It's going to be so nice to see my sister and her family next week- I've really missed them."

4. **Share a request you have of your partner.** There may be times when you truly do not have anything to request, but you are strongly encouraged to try to come up with something. Examples:
   - "It would mean a lot to me if you could remember to pick up your socks and underwear from the floor before you go to work."
   - "Every time you call me from work it helps me feel loved and appreciated- please keep doing that!"
   - "I know I've asked this before, but I'd really like you to hear me this time...I need you to stop talking about our money problems in front of the kids. Could you please promise to wait until we have privacy to have those discussions?"

Shared Commitment Planned Intimate Experience:

Couples Recovery Check-In
(Bercaw & Bercaw)

Purpose and Goals:

One of the challenges in restoring trust during the recovery process involves managing the flow of recovery information. This PIE is designed to ensure that the proper information is flowing and that it is flowing in the right direction. That direction always is initiated from recovering addict to recovering spouse. This keeps the spouse out of the "nag" or "police" roles that no one ever aspires to hold. Because the Recovery Check-In (RCI) occurs on a regular schedule, many spouses experience that it helps them manage some of their typical anxieties. For instance, when a question or worry comes to mind, there is comfort in knowing that in just a few days there will be a natural time to address it. Likewise, the recovering addict often benefits from feeling secure in knowing when s/he will be sharing specific recovery information (or being asked for it) instead of feeling "ambushed" with questions. Recovering addicts using this format can share themselves in a way that is integrity-based, moderate and forthcoming. Finally, this process works best when the recovering spouse is able to share about his/her recovery, promoting a spirit of mutuality.

Instructions:

First, a foundation needs to be established: Each person writes out what their recovery program looks like. Use the categories below to make sure you are covering the basics:

1. Bottom line behaviors: (those that I've promised "never again," and would require me to re-start my sobriety count)
2. Recovery Action Steps/Program Practice: (12-step meeting schedule, frequency of sponsor contact, individual/couples/group therapy, phone calls, meditation, prayer, recovery reading, etc.)

Schedule a time to walk each other through your recovery program. This is not done so that spouses can evaluate or manage each other's programs, but simply to provide clarity on basic recovery information. It may, however, be a time to ask questions (e.g. "I'm confused because I thought you had said before that you were talking to your sponsor daily, but just now you said 'often.' Could you please clarify that for me?")

After reviewing your programs, you are positioned to complete the RCI Contract (on the following page). Be sure that you are meeting for RCI's at least once a month, but no more than once a week. Also be sure to negotiate the level of detail desired regarding slips in sobriety. Your therapist may be helpful in processing questions around appropriate levels of detail.

Recovery Check-In Contract

(Bercaw & Bercaw)

We are mutually committed to being active in our individual and couples recoveries. This contract formalizes our commitment to regularly share with each other about recovery.

We commit to meet every ____ weeks (on _____ at _____ o'clock)

Note: If one spouse is unavailable for a regularly scheduled RCI, it is that spouse's responsibility to suggest a make-up date at the earliest possible time.

The following are possible topics for sharing. Review this list together and negotiate specific items for each of your check-ins:

- Sobriety status (note slips/relapse if applicable)
- Recovery work completed
- Most helpful recovery step since last check-in
- Least useful behavior since last RCI
- Emotional state(s) since last RCI
- Physical state(s) since last RCI
- Spiritual state(s) since last RCI
- Ongoing or upcoming stressors (and need for help)
- Upcoming hopes and aspirations

Choose from the list above and supplement with any of your own mutually agreed upon topics. Then write these topics in the space provided below.

When I check-in I will share about:

How it works: Once you have agreed to the specific times and topics, you are ready to transition to the *ongoing process of Recovery Check-In*. A typical RCI involves:

a) Recovering addict initiates at the agreed upon time and shares his/her RCI

b) Recovering spouse shares his/her RCI

c) Each person asks any questions they may have in response to the other's RCI or questions they may have been saving for this specific time

d) In the spirit of Recovering Couples Anonymous (RCA), each person shares something they have done since last RCI that has NOT been helpful to their spouse and also shares something their spouse has done that HAS been helpful.

By signing below, we agree to abide by this contract.

| _____ | | _____ | |
| Name | Date | Name | Date |

Shared Commitment Planned Intimate Experience:

Past, Present and Future
(Bercaw & Bercaw)

<u>**Instructions:**</u>

Please reflect on the following aspects of your relationship in terms of the way you have experienced them in the past, the way you experience them in the present and the way you hope to experience them in the future. Then get together with your spouse during your PIE time to share your responses. Remember that you are sharing to be known better by your spouse, and listening so you may know your spouse better.

Example: 3. Trust: "In the past, I trusted my spouse implicitly with everything. Presently, I really struggle to trust him in certain areas, like spending and following through on his promises. But I hope to be able to experience more trust in these departments in the future. I think it is normal to have some areas in a shared relationship where the trust level varies."

1. *Emotional closeness*

2. *Spiritual Connection*

3. *Trust*

4. *Communication*

5. *Dependability*

6. *Fun/Joy Together*

7. *Romantic Passion*

8. *Negotiating Compromise*

Shared Commitment Planned Intimate Experience:

A View from the Top
(Bercaw & Bercaw)

Purpose and Goals:

This PIE is designed to consolidate your "future" responses from the *Past, Present, Future* PIE into a vision for the relationship you want to enjoy with each other. This vision is a key component of couples' healing. You need to see clearly how you would *like* to be in relationship in order to work toward getting there. This PIE will also give you a window into how your spouse imagines the best version of your relationship.

Instructions:

Review your responses from the "Future" portions of the "Past, Present and Future" PIE you recently completed. Allow your mind to imagine a time when you are enjoying a much improved way of experiencing your relationship. Imagine that you are looking at all that you have and you are connecting with the gratitude that is there. You see noticeable shifts that have been made, both inside and outside the bedroom. You see pain that has been transformed. You see a version of yourself that you really like. See how you are able to be true to yourself in your relationship. You see how you are able to freely and fully enjoy sexual intimacy and all of its possibilities. You see yourself experiencing more and more pleasure, comfort, presence and joy with your spouse. Allow yourself to see all of this and to feel whatever is there. When you have a clear image of this and a good connection with the accompanying feelings, write about it: Describe what you see from this "mountaintop." Consider the following:

- What does your facial expression and body language look like?

- What about your spouse's?

- What kinds of activities do you see yourselves doing?

- How do you feel about yourself in this relationship?

- What is different about what you see in this relationship?

- What have you chosen to retain from your past/present in this relationship?

- What feelings do you notice as you envision this relationship?

Share your reflections with your spouse during your scheduled PIE time.

10

Phase II: Courageous Discovery

Having built momentum around your emotional intimacy in the previous chapter, you will be focusing more on the physical and sensual aspects of your intimacy in the Courageous Discovery phase. Each of you will be asked to identify the sexual attitudes and automatic thoughts you have brought to the relationship, and to explore how those attitudes have interacted with your relationship dynamics. Sharing your enhanced awareness will pull for feelings of vulnerability. The structure of the PIEs is intended to provide a safe framework for you to risk that vulnerability. Each time that you do, your intimacy grows and the potential for a new passion grows with it.

This is the stage when the first caressing experiences are introduced. You may be surprised at the strong emotions that surface when giving and receiving this slow, sensual type of touch. Your emotions are experienced as a function of your ability to be present. Presence is the polar opposite of living with addiction, in which behavior is unconsciously geared toward avoidance. This phase of SRT represents a concrete opportunity to take healthy ownership of your *sensuality* by experiencing touch in a way that is characterized by more presence than ever before. As each of you embraces the idea that you are responsible for your own pleasure and you are encouraged to ask for what you need and want, you will be laying the foundation for the healthy sexual intimacy you want. Part of that process involves challenging and discarding outdated ways of thinking about yourselves and your sexuality. This phase is all about openness to new experiences and the discoveries they yield. It is about gathering the courage to share your discoveries so that your intimacy may grow.

Mutual Agreements: Courageous Discovery
(Bercaw & Bercaw)

Instructions:

Read the following statements aloud and together and place your initials in the space provided next to each one to indicate your agreement. (If you are not sure that you agree, please circle the statement so you remember to discuss it with your therapist at your next meeting.)

1. We agree to search ourselves in order to identify old sexual beliefs and feelings. Then we will be able to decide which ones to keep and which to discard. _____

2. We agree to risk sharing our growing insights as we become aware of them, even when we become aware of difficulties or painful realities. _____

3. We agree to be respectful of any uncomfortable feelings that may be experienced during this time by each other. _____

4. We commit to embracing a spirit of compassion and empathy as we connect with our woundedness and our imperfections. _____

5. We commit to a good faith effort to try some new ways of enjoying sensual touch. _____

Courageous Discovery
Action Steps

- Examine sexual beliefs, identify intimacy obstacles
- Embrace vulnerability
- Share new self-awareness with each other to enhance intimacy
- Begin to claim your own healthy sexuality
- Communicate warmth/nurturance through touch
- Ask for what you prefer; welcome being asked

Courageous Discovery Planned Intimate Experience:

Hands and Feet Pleasuring
(Bercaw & Bercaw)

Purpose and Goals:
    This PIE is designed to allow you to enjoy a new type of sensual touch and to enjoy your introduction to the roles of caresser and receiver. Caressing and having one's hands and feet caressed can be surprisingly comforting and connecting. It begins the process of expanding your capacity to slow things down and to appreciate a wider range of sensual pleasure than may have been the case up until this point. The environment is carefully set up to be free of demand or expectations of any kind. The emphasis is on experimenting with a new type of touch within the context of the structure provided in the instructions below.

Instructions: [18]
    This experience can occur wherever you think would be the most comfortable (such as a couch, bed, or chair). You will be taking turns caressing and being caressed. The areas of the body that will be caressed are the hands and feet. The initiator sets up the room in a way that feels honoring of the experience to come. Then, the initiator communicates that the room is set up and ready.

    Once both people are in the room, the person who has agreed to be the first receiver assumes a comfortable position and then tells the caresser that s/he is ready. As the caresser, begin by asking your spouse whether hands or feet would be best to start with. Then begin to lightly caress that part of the body. Let your enjoyment of your spouse's body guide your caressing. You can assume that your spouse is enjoying the caress unless you hear otherwise. It is the receiver's responsibility to communicate a preference for the caresser to change the type of touch or location of the touch. When either the caresser or receiver wants to transition to the next part of the body (whatever has not been caressed yet), simply communicate this preference. Likewise, whenever it occurs to either spouse that they have had enough time caressing or being caressed (after the receiver's hands AND feet have been caressed), this should be expressed as well. Then you can switch roles (receiver becomes caresser, caresser becomes receiver).

    As the caresser, you are free to enjoy and appreciate being trusted with your spouse's body. As the receiver, you are free to enjoy and appreciate being the focus of your spouse's warm and loving caress. However, if either of you experiences anxiety that interferes with being present and engaged in the experience, it is your responsibility to say so. If this happens, it may be wise to take a break and then re-evaluate how best to continue. Options include: Making adjustments to help the experience feel more comfortable; or agreeing to stop the touching part of the experience and transition to recording the experience in your journals.

***

When each of you has had enough time caressing, it is time to record your thoughts and feelings about this experience in your journals. (What did you enjoy the most? Would you choose to do this again, and if so, would you want to make any modifications? Did you encounter any barriers? What feelings were you aware of? How would you describe your comfort level? What are your feelings toward your spouse?)

Note: This experience is not designed to be inherently arousing. If either of you becomes aroused, that is fine, but it is certainly not the goal. It is important to surrender any *pursuit and/or monitoring of arousal* in order to allow yourselves to be optimally present with each other and to maintain optimal awareness of all that you are experiencing.

Courageous Discovery Planned Intimate Experience:

Self Image Assessment
(Bercaw & Bercaw)

Purpose and Goals:

This PIE will help you identify self-perceptions and feelings about your body. It provides an opportunity to share these self-perceptions and feelings with your spouse, and to be a safe person for your spouse during his/her sharing. This exercise may be somewhat challenging, as many people feel uncomfortable connecting with the feelings they have about their physical selves. It is for this reason that it presents an excellent opportunity to know your spouse more fully and to allow yourself to be more fully known. This is how we cultivate intimacy. You can set boundaries with your spouse before, during and after this exercise in order to feel safe (e.g. telling your spouse that you feel nervous and would prefer that s/he take the first turn).

Instructions

Fill out the following sentence completion items on your own and then schedule a time with your spouse to share your responses. When you are both done sharing and discussing, make notes at the bottom of this page regarding how it felt to share what you did and what it was like to hear your spouse share.

1. The part of my body I feel best about is my_____ because _____
2. The part of my body I feel worst about is my _____ because _____
3. In my mind I imagine that when you see my body you think, "_____"
4. (Men) I have always thought that my penis is_____
5. (Women) I have always thought that my vagina is _____
6. When you see me naked I feel_____
7. When I was younger, I felt most secure about my _____
8. When I was younger, I felt most insecure about my _____
9. I had the most positive feelings about my body when I was ___ years old because…
10. I had the most negative feelings about my body when I was ___ years old because…
11. The part of my body that has changed the most through the years is my _____
12. The part of my body I'm most concerned about as I think about getting older is my _____.
13. Something I could be doing differently to feel better about my body is _____.
14. The part of your body I like the best is your _____ (and a close second would be your _____).

91

Courageous Discovery Planned Intimate Experience:

Face
(Bercaw & Bercaw)

Purpose and Goals:

This PIE (Planned Intimate Experience) is intended to provide you with a uniquely connecting opportunity. Whenever you think about your spouse, the image of his/her face automatically comes into your mind. In our daily lives, we may shake hands, give a pat on the back, or even place a supportive hand on someone's shoulder. But the face is much different; when we allow someone to touch our face it is deeply personal. To invite your spouse to do this is a very intimate gesture. As the receiver, you allow yourself to be vulnerable. As the caresser, you can be respectful of the gift of your spouse's vulnerability. Whenever you choose to be vulnerability together your shared intimacy is deepened.

Instructions:[19]

This experience can occur wherever you think would be most comfortable (couch, bed, chair, blanket on the floor, etc). You will take turns caressing and being caressed. The specific area of the body that will be caressed is the face (including head, hair, ears and neck). The initiator sets up the room in a way that feels honoring of the experience to come. Then, the initiator communicates that the room is set up and ready.

Once both people are in the room, the person who has agreed to be the first receiver finds a comfortable position and tells the caresser that s/he is ready. As the caresser, begin by lightly caressing your spouse's face, head, hair, ears and neck. Let your enjoyment of your spouse's body guide your touch. Assume that the receiver is enjoying the caress unless you hear otherwise. As the receiver, remember to communicate any preferences for a different kind of touch. Whenever it occurs to either of you that you have had enough time caressing or being caressed, express that you are ready to switch roles (receiver becomes caresser, caresser becomes receiver).

As the caresser, you can enjoy and appreciate being trusted with your spouse's body. As the receiver, you can enjoy and appreciate being the focus of your spouse's warm and loving caress. However, if either of you experiences anxiety that interferes with being present and engaged in the experience, it is your responsibility to say so. If this happens, it may be wise to take a break and then re-evaluate how to continue. Options include: Making adjustments to help the experience feel more comfortable; switching roles; limiting the touch to one specific area that is most comfortable; or agreeing to stop the touching part of the experience and transition to recording the experience in your journals.

***

When both of you have had enough caress time, it is time to record your thoughts and feelings about this PIE in your journals. (What did you enjoy the most? Would you choose to do this again, and if so, would you want to make any modifications? Did you encounter any barriers? What feelings were you aware of? How would you describe your comfort level? What are your feelings of closeness toward your spouse?) When you are both done writing, share what you have written with each other.

Note: This experience is not designed to be inherently arousing. If either spouse becomes aroused, that is fine, but it is certainly not the goal. It is important to surrender any *pursuit and/or monitoring of arousal* in order to allow yourselves to be optimally present with each other and to maintain optimal awareness of all that you are experiencing.

Note: Some people are very uncomfortable with others touching their face. If this is the case for either one of you, discuss how you might modify the experience to work around this sensitivity (e.g. focus mostly on the head, hair, ears and neck)

Courageous Discovery Planned Intimate Experience:

The Other Side of the Door
(Bercaw & Bercaw)

Purpose and Goals:

When we talk about intimacy, we are really referring to the process of being known by another person and also of knowing that person. Intimacy involves sharing oneself in an honest and real way and being open to another person's authentic sharing as well. It is a two-way street. If you are reading this book, chances are that there has been some ongoing tension around intimacy. This PIE creates a unique experience to help you look at this most fundamental component of relationships and work toward making it more comfortable. It is absolutely possible to develop more skills and comfort in this area by working at it. This PIE is designed to allow you to connect with the tension that often exists between desiring more intimacy and the barriers to experiencing that intimacy.

Instructions:

This experience will occur around a door (bedroom, bathroom, closet – any of these will do). Choose a time when you are assured to have privacy and when the house is most quiet such as after the children are asleep. One of you can bring a timer to the room and set it for a period of time to which you both agree (10 minutes or so can be enough, but feel free to do more). Have your journals in hand before beginning.

You are asked to close the bedroom door with each of you on opposite sides of it. Next, sit down with your legs crossed and tucked underneath you (some call this "Indian Style"). Try to get your knees as close to the door as possible. As you breathe deeply and sit in silence, try to visualize your spouse on the other side. Focus on the image you have of your spouse on the other side; your spouse's eyes, nose, lips, ears, facial expression, and demeanor. You may wish to gently place your hands on the door's surface once you have been able to focus on the visualization. Allow yourself to notice the silence and stillness of this moment. Notice whatever feelings are there. Connect with your breathing as you connect with what you are feeling. If you notice your mind drifting, this is not unusual; simply try to refocus if this happens. Keep breathing, visualizing, noticing and feeling until the timer tells you to stop.

***

Before reconnecting with your spouse, go immediately to your journal and record all that you can about this experience. What feelings and thoughts were you aware of? What did you visualize about your spouse on the other side? To what extent were you able to stay present? Did you experience any obstacles or distractions?

Wait until you are both done writing, then open the door and embrace your spouse with a hug. Now it is time to share your responses.

Courageous Discovery Planned Intimate Experience:

Mutual Gaze
(Bercaw & Bercaw)

Purpose and Goals:

As you continue to focus on enhancing your intimacy, this PIE gives you the chance to do so in a rather novel setting. This PIE is to be done soon after you have completed "The Other Side of The Door." While that PIE facilitated the experience of being separate yet connected, this PIE removes the physical barrier of the door. It allows another way to connect intimately with each other while maintaining a gaze directly into your spouse's eyes. Research has demonstrated a very strong correlation between looking directly into someone's eyes and having increased positive feelings for that person.

The experience of gazing deeply into a lover's eyes is romanticized in movies and TV. However, this is not a naturally comfortable experience for many of us. In fact, it can be a situation in which we feel quite vulnerable. If that is true for you, you may feel a little bit "naked" outside the bedroom in this PIE. Why? The eyes are both our windows to our souls as well as access to the souls of others. As such, extended eye contact is loaded with the potential for big feelings.

You have attempted many new behaviors throughout your recoveries and have become vastly more competent in many new areas. The goal here is not to become more comfortable with eye contact with everyone, but simply to increase your comfort and presence with your spouse.

Instructions:

This experience can occur in any room of your house that is peaceful and private. If it is your turn to initiate, set up the room in a way that feels honoring of the experience and bring a timer to the room. Just before beginning the experience, set the timer for a period of time to which you both agree (3-5 minutes or so can be enough for your first time).

You are asked to sit facing each other. If it is physically comfortable, you can sit down with your legs crossed and tucked underneath you (like in the previous PIE). Try to get your knees as close to your spouse's knees as possible. Start the timer.

If comfortable, allow your hands to rest gently on top of or underneath your spouse's hands. Breathe deeply as you begin looking into your spouse's eyes. Focus on your breathing so you may be as present as possible. Please resist the temptation to giggle or to try to make your spouse laugh; it may be what feels natural, but will distract from the experience of allowing you to be fully present.

Allow yourself to *see* your spouse. Of course you see him/her right there in front of you, but can you also see the courage and vulnerability in those eyes? What else do you see in those eyes? Fear? Joy? Kindness? Trust? Sadness? Try to be mindful of the fact that those are the same eyes through which your spouse saw the world long before the two of you ever met. Do you see the person you originally fell in love with? Do you see the person you choose to love every day?

95

Embrace the silence and stillness of this moment. Notice whatever it is that you are feeling. Stay focused on your breathing as you connect with what you are feeling. If you notice your mind drifting, simply try to refocus. Keep gazing, noticing and feeling until the timer tells you to stop. (You may choose to end this experience by embracing your spouse with a hug, if that is what you both want).

***

Go immediately to your journal and record all that you can about this experience. What feelings and thoughts were you aware of? To what extent were you able to stay present? Did you experience any obstacles or distractions? What was comfortable about this time together? What was uncomfortable? What messages were you given about making eye contact when you were growing up? Was this viewed as positive or negative in your family of origin?

When you are both done writing, share your responses.

Courageous Discovery Planned Intimate Experience:

Back
(Bercaw & Bercaw)

Purpose and Goals:

This PIE is designed to allow you to enjoy the new type of touch you are learning, this time on another area of the body. This experience focuses on your back. Many people have experience in giving or receiving a back *massage*. Here, you are asked to experiment with a lighter type of touch than a traditional massage in order to elevate the intimacy potential. Rather than simply relieving muscle tension, gently caressing the back in this experience allows each spouse to feel closely connected through the touch. There is more surface area to cover on the back than on your previous caressing exercises, and you are encouraged to explore the sensual and emotional potential that various parts of this area may hold. You are continuing to grow your capacity to slow things down and to appreciate a wider range of sensual pleasure than may have been the case up until this point. The environment is carefully set up to be free of demand or expectations of any kind. The emphasis is on experimenting with a new type of touch within the context of the structure provided in the instructions below.

Instructions:[20]

This experience can occur wherever you think would be the most comfortable. Again, you will take turns caressing and being caressed. The area that will be caressed is the back. This includes everything from the base of the neck down to the hips. The initiator sets up the room in a way that feels honoring of the experience to come. Then, the initiator communicates that the room is set up and ready.

As the receiver, you are free to choose the amount of clothing you prefer while being caressed. Some people may choose to be completely naked, while others may prefer to wear underwear, a t-shirt, or pajamas. There is no right or wrong attire for this exercise, as long as you both are comfortable. You may each choose to be in different states of undress while receiving. Once both people are in the room, the person who has agreed to be the first receiver takes a position that feels comfortable while lying face down, then communicates to the caresser that s/he is ready.

As the caresser, you are free to enjoy the experience of caressing your spouse's back. Let your enjoyment of your spouse's body guide your touch. You can assume that your spouse is enjoying the touch unless s/he redirects you. You can be aware of the nuances of your spouse's back, and can appreciate being trusted with your spouse's vulnerability. As the receiver, you can be aware of how the touch feels different as it moves from one region to another. You might also appreciate the careful attention that the caresser is demonstrating. Whenever it occurs to either of you that you have had enough time caressing or being caressed this should be expressed. Then you can switch roles (receiver becomes caresser, caresser becomes receiver).

If either of you experiences any anxiety that begins to interfere with being present and engaged in the experience, it is that person's responsibility to communicate this. At this point it may be wise to take a break and re-evaluate and discuss how to proceed. Options include making adjustments to help the experience feel more comfortable or agreeing to stop the touching part of the experience and transition to recording the experience in your journals.

***

When both of you have had enough time caressing, it is time to record your thoughts and feelings about this experience in your journals. (What did you enjoy the most? Would you choose to do this again? If so, would you want to make any modifications? Did you encounter any barriers? What feelings were you aware of? How would you describe your comfort level? What are your feelings toward your spouse right now?)

Note: This experience is not designed to be inherently arousing. If either spouse becomes aroused, that may be a positive experience, but it is not the goal. It is important to surrender any *pursuit and/or monitoring of arousal* in order to allow yourselves to be optimally present with each other and to maintain optimal awareness of everything that you are experiencing.

Courageous Discovery Planned Intimate Experience:

Mirror, Mirror
(Bercaw & Bercaw)

Purpose and Goals:
You know that when you share a vulnerable moment with your spouse, you tend to feel closer and more bonded. One common area of vulnerability relates to our physical bodies. This PIE is designed to help you to be vulnerable with your spouse in a contained way. Specifically, you will strive to be present with your thoughts and feelings about your bodies.

Most spouses differ in the ways they feel about their bodies. Usually one person has more positive feelings about his/her own body and one has more negative feelings. This PIE gives both of you an opportunity to share your feelings honestly and to continue to develop greater levels of trust and empathy for each other. In this way, you are not only revealing your bodies to each other, but some true feelings as well.

Some people experience anxiety as they approach and participate in this PIE. This can be especially true if you have been guarded with your body in the wake of a disclosure or discovery. Again, you will have an opportunity to share your reality with your spouse and ask for some understanding around your discomfort. Much can be gained from the interactions that occur before and after the PIEs regardless of what actually happens during the PIEs.

Instructions:[21]
This experience requires a mirror (preferably full-length). If one person is less comfortable with this PIE, then that person should be responsible for setting up the room. In this way s/he can adjust the lighting and temperature and other variables to enhance his/her comfort. Eventually, the hope is that both spouses will be comfortable completing this PIE while naked, but it is fine if you are not able to start there. Some people may choose to be completely naked for their initial experience with this PIE, while others may prefer to wear underwear, a t-shirt, or pajamas. There is no right or wrong attire for this exercise, as long as you both are comfortable. In fact, you each may choose to be in different states of undress.

Whoever goes first is asked to stand in front of the mirror. Take a deep, centering breath and then share how you feel about each part of your body. Start at the top of your head and go all the way down to your toes, not skipping anything in between. Please be as specific as possible in your monologue. For example, instead of just addressing your "face," please share your feelings about your hair, ears, eyes, teeth, lips smile, nose, eyebrows, and chin. And even if you do choose to wear some clothing, please share your feelings about the parts of your body that are covered by the clothing. All the while, the person who is not in front of the mirror is sitting off to the side, simply listening with full attention and appreciation for your spouse's willingness to share what they are sharing right now.

Sometimes, how we feel about a part of our body changes over time. Please mention if this happens to be the case for any part of your body (e.g. "I used to like my hair when I had more of it;" or "I thought my eyes were really pretty until I started to get these crows' feet")

When the first person has finished, the spouse who has been listening should offer a summary of what s/he has just heard and can offer supportive feedback that is genuine. (For example: "It sounds like you're pretty comfortable with your body in general, except for your "X" and your "Y." To tell you the truth, I've always kind of liked your "X" and your "Y." I know how insecure you've been feeling about your "Y" for a long time, and I hope you find a way to make peace with yourself. Thank you for walking me through everything you just did. I know that wasn't easy for you."). At this point, you are asked to switch roles and go through the same process as above.

***

When you have completed the experience, take a moment to reflect on what it was like for you and record your reflections in your journal. What themes did you notice about your thoughts and feelings about your body? How would you describe your comfort level? Did it vary according to what part of your body you were commenting on? What did you sense from your spouse when s/he was sharing? How about when your spouse was listening and then giving you feedback?

Please share the notes you made with each other and *know that you have shared a significant accomplishment in what you just did together.*

Courageous Discovery Planned Intimate Experience:

Sensual Bathing
(Bercaw & Bercaw)

Purpose and Goals:

This PIE is intended to allow you to enjoy each other's bodies in a sensual setting. Taking a bath or shower together is something you may already be familiar with. However, this PIE is designed to be qualitatively different from your previous experiences. You may notice from the previous caressing PIEs that when you slow things down your experience is affected. Here, you are again asked to slow down, and you may find that your experience of your spouse, yourself, and perhaps your environment is affected. You may continue to notice and appreciate some aspects of your spouse and yourself that may not have been apparent before. This is designed to be primarily a *sensual* experience and not just for washing up. The goal is to remain open to the newness of this experience as you continue to expand your menu of pleasurable activities.

Instructions:[22]

This experience can occur in a bathtub or shower (wherever you think would be most comfortable). You will take turns washing and caressing each other. While you may choose to be naked for this experience, it is important to use the "Bikini Rule" at this stage. This means that anything that would be covered by a bikini (breasts, genitals) is not yet included in the washing or caressing. The initiator sets up the bathroom in a way that feels honoring of the experience to come. Then, the initiator communicates that the room is set up and ready.

Once both of you are present you can enter the tub/shower. It is important that each person choose the amount of clothing that is most comfortable to them. For example, one spouse may choose to be naked while the other wishes to wear a swimsuit. It is sometimes the case that one spouse would be most comfortable if *both* were to wear swimsuits. If you do choose some clothing, just know that eventually and as gradually as you are comfortable the goal will be to experience this PIE while both of you are naked.

Once in the tub/shower, the person who has agreed to be the first receiver finds a position that feels comfortable, then communicates to the caresser that s/he is ready. As the caresser, you are then free to wash and caress your spouse's hair and body. Let your enjoyment of your spouse's body guide your touch. You can assume that your spouse is enjoying the washing and caressing unless you hear otherwise. As the receiver, remember to communicate any preferences you have for your spouse to change the type or location of the touch. Whenever either spouse is ready to switch roles, this should be expressed. When either spouse would like to exit the tub/shower, this should also be communicated. Then you are free to dry each other with a comfortable towel, again being mindful of the Bikini Rule.

If either of you experiences any anxiety that interferes with being present and engaged in the experience, it is that person's responsibility to communicate this. At this point it may be wise to take a break to re-evaluate and discuss how to proceed. Options include making adjustments to help the experience feel more comfortable (switching roles, limiting the touch to one specific area that is most comfortable) or agreeing to stop the touching part of the experience and transition to recording the experience in your journals.

***

When each of you has had enough washing and caressing, it is time to record your thoughts and feelings about this experience in your journals. (What did you enjoy the most? Would you choose to do this again, and if so, would you want to make any modifications? Did you encounter any barriers? What feelings were you aware of? How would you describe your comfort level? What are your feelings toward your spouse?)

Note: This experience is not designed to be inherently arousing. If either spouse becomes aroused, that is fine, but it is not the goal. It is important to surrender any *pursuit and/or monitoring of arousal* in order to allow yourselves to be optimally present with each other and to maintain optimal awareness of all that you are experiencing.

Courageous Discovery Planned Intimate Experience:

Quiet Cuddle
(Bercaw &Bercaw)

Purpose and Goals:

This PIE is intended to provide another safe atmosphere for each of you to enjoy physical closeness. This feeling of safety is something that you may not have experienced in your past physical encounters, and each of you may have different experiences of it now as well. This PIE gives the spouse who tends to feel less safe and more anxious a way to gradually establish and build upon a new foundation of safety and trust. It also gives the spouse who tends naturally to feel safer an opportunity to demonstrate compassion and to be receptive to his/her spouse's safety needs. The environment is carefully set up to be free of demands. The emphasis is on experiencing relaxation while in the close physical presence of your spouse.

Instructions:

This experience can occur anywhere you are comfortable (in bed, on the couch, or a blanket on the floor). The initiator sets up the room in a way that feels honoring of the experience. Then, the initiator communicates that the room is set up and ready.

Once both people are in the room, the person who tends to experience the most anxiety around physical encounters gets onto the bed/couch first and gets comfortable (If neither of you tends to have any discomfort or anxiety around physical intimacy, just flip a coin!) For the purpose of this PIE, that person will be in the receiver role. As the receiver, you can invite your spouse to join you once you feel centered and present. For the purpose of this PIE, the person being invited is the caresser. As the caresser, you can slowly approach your spouse until you are close enough to gently get into a "spooning" position. Together, you can quietly maintain this position for a time that feels comfortable to both. It is important to stay as present with each other and with oneself as possible, being aware of your body and as many senses as possible. What does the pillow feel like against your head? Can you feel the warmth of your spouse's body next to yours? Are there any scents or sounds you are aware of? Try to also notice your emotions. Are you feeling nervous, relaxed, joyful, guilty, ashamed, love, sad?

After of period of holding this position, either of you may express when you are ready to switch roles (receiver becomes caresser, caresser becomes receiver). If you become emotionally or physically uncomfortable at any time and would benefit from making an adjustment, it is important that you share this with your spouse.

***

Whenever either spouse has had enough cuddling, you may communicate this and move on to the final part of this exercise, *recording* your experience in your journal. Take a moment to record some of the thoughts and feelings you just experienced. What was this like for you? What did you enjoy? What was challenging? Would you choose to do this again? If so, would you make any modifications?

Courageous Discovery Planned Intimate Experience:

Body Caressing (excluding breasts and genitals)
(Bercaw & Bercaw)

Purpose and Goals:

This PIE is a combination of the previous caressing PIEs you have completed. In this PIE, you are going to be able to enjoy caressing and being caressed over you entire bodies, with the exception of the breasts and genitals (the "Bikini Rule" still applies). There is more freedom to explore and enjoy each others' bodies with the new type of caressing touch you have been experimenting with. Again, you are encouraged to explore the sensual and emotional potential that various areas of your bodies may hold. You are continuing to grow your capacity to slow things down and appreciate a broad range of sensual pleasure.

The environment is set up to be free of demand or expectations of any kind. Nevertheless, it may be challenging for some people to respect the boundaries of the Bikini Rule and for others to trust that the boundaries will be respected. It may be helpful to understand that the purpose of the Bikini Rule is to keep things safe, predictable and contained. It also promotes staying connected with what you *have* in the present moment, which hopefully is a very pleasurable touch experience. Most spouses are less familiar with some of the satisfying appetizers available on the menu of pleasurable touch than they are with the main entrées! In PIEs such as this one, you are building up the menu items available to you in your shared sensual and sexual relationship. In fact, you might find that the appetizers you have skipped over before now make the entrees even *more* satisfying. If you do have concerns about the Bikini Rule, you should share your concerns at this time with your spouse.

Finally, you are continuing to develop awareness of your own touch preferences. You are also learning to trust that sharing your preferences is (or is becoming) a safe thing to do. You continue to remain open to any such feedback or redirection from your spouse, understanding that such communications are themselves, acts of intimacy.

Instructions:[23]

This experience is probably best suited for a room or area in your home where you can be comfortable lying down (bed, couch, blanket on floor). You will be taking turns caressing and being caressed over the entire body with the exception of the breasts and genitals. The initiator sets up the room in a way that feels honoring of the experience to come. Then, the initiator communicates that the room is set up and ready. *You will begin by enjoying a sensual time of bathing or showering together, just as you did in the Sensual Bathing PIE.* It will now be customary to begin your caressing PIEs by bathing or showering together. (Because this is a prelude to other PIEs now, it is perfectly acceptable to have a more brief time of bathing/showering than in the Sensual Bathing PIE).

After enjoying the bath or shower time, the first receiver is free to choose the amount of clothing s/he prefers while being caressed. As the receiver, you may choose to be completely naked, or to wear some light clothing (underwear, a t-shirt, or pajamas). There is no right or wrong attire for this, as long as you both are comfortable. In fact, you each may choose to be in different states of undress while receiving. If you choose some amount of clothing, just know that eventually and as gradually as you are comfortable the goal will be to experience this PIE while both of you are naked.

As the receiver, find a position that feels comfortable while lying face down, then communicate to the caresser that you are ready. Be mindful of any touch preferences you are aware of while being caressed and verbalize them to your spouse. As the caresser, you are free to begin enjoying the experience of caressing the back of your spouse's body, from head to toe. Remember to assume that your spouse is enjoying the touch unless s/he redirects you.

Whenever it occurs to the RECEIVER that s/he is ready to have the front of his/her body caressed, this should be stated. After of period of caressing the front of the body, either of you may express when you are ready to switch roles (receiver becomes caresser, caresser becomes receiver).

If either of you experiences anxiety that interferes with being present and engaged in the experience, it is best to communicate this. At this point it may be wise to take a break and then re-evaluate and discuss how to proceed. Options include making adjustments to help the experience feel more comfortable or agreeing to stop the touching part of the experience and transition to recording the experience in your journals.

* * *

When both of you have had enough caressing, it is time to record your thoughts and feelings about this experience in your journals or in the space below. (What did you enjoy the most? Would you choose to do this again, and if so, would you want to make any modifications? Did you encounter any barriers? What feelings were you aware of? How would you describe your comfort level? What are your feelings toward your spouse?)

Note: This experience is not designed to be inherently arousing. If either spouse becomes aroused, that is fine, but it is not the goal. It is important to surrender any *pursuit and/or monitoring of arousal* in order to allow yourselves to be optimally present with each other and to maintain optimal awareness of all that you are experiencing.

Courageous Discovery Planned Intimate Experience:

Front Door/Side Door
(Bercaw & Bercaw)

Purpose and Goals:

Everyone has needs and wants. But many of us have a long history of difficulty getting our needs and wants met in relationships. This is one of the hallmarks of what is known as *codependence*. It is common for both addicts and spouses to have some codependent traits and to take an indirect or "side door" approach to their needs and wants. This approach lends itself to resentment and/or secrecy. On the other hand, using a respectful and direct "front door" approach is both empowering and intimacy-building. The front door leads to personal integrity and enhanced trust. *Couple's recovery is all about choosing to knock on the front door, despite a well-worn and familiar path to the side door.* The following communication PIE is designed to help you identify the ways in which you tend toward indirect approaches (Side Door) and to see how you can work toward more direct (Front Door) approaches.

Side Door:

The indirect approach involves not sharing clearly your needs or wants with your spouse. Often, there is a fear that any such sharing would be met with rejection or would be criticized or diminished. Part of this fear may be based on your history with the spouse, but some of this fear was likely learned long before you ever knew each other. The result is that in certain moments you see your spouse as a threat and fear his/her response to sharing your needs and wants. This often occurs seamlessly on an unconscious level. It is simply how you act and react in your default mode.

Think about times when you have used an indirect approach when you wanted or needed something. Did you make yourself obviously helpless hoping that help would be offered? (e.g. trying to carry more groceries than you could manage; shivering if you wanted the heat turned up) Did you deny or minimize what you needed? (e.g. "It's not a big deal, I'll be fine.") Did you remain silent, never sharing what you wanted? Or perhaps you just did what you wanted without involving your spouse at all, and kept it a secret. (e.g. making a purchase or investment). Even when we get our way, these indirect techniques keep us stuck and powerless. They reinforce the inaccurate beliefs that a) your spouse is someone to be feared and b) that you will not be able to tolerate a negative response (if there is one).

Some will say, "But I have no problem being direct- I always let people know where I stand." This gets tricky, because some people *can* be very straightforward in many areas of their lives (e.g. professional), but reserve the side door for other areas (e.g. asking for help). There is usually at pocket of indirectness that resides in us all. The challenge is to search for yours.

After reading the samples below, list three "Side Door" examples of your own:

106

SAMPLE #1: When you ask me to help with something and it's really not a good time for me, I often say yes anyway. Then I feel annoyed with you and start to distance myself. I feel unappreciated for helping you when it was inconvenient for me, but I never told you it was inconvenient in the first place. Sometimes this will happen over and over, with me feeling unappreciated and resentful until finally I snap at you. Then I make myself feel guilty.

SAMPLE #2: I need more help getting the kids ready for school in the morning, but don't ask you because you seem stressed and angry and I don't want to set you off. But I end up stressed and angry too when I feel like I'm on my own to make lunches, get them dressed, make breakfast, brush their teeth and get myself ready too. I make myself feel helpless and on my own even when you are in the same room with me.

SAMPLE #3: When you said you wanted to paint our room lavender and I went along with it, even though I didn't want that color. I feel like I can't say what I want ever since I got busted. So I end up making myself feel angry at you because I have to live with this purple room.

SAMPLE #4: When we are deciding what to have for dinner and I'll say, "I don't care, what do *you* want?" But sometimes I do care and I hold back from saying what my preference is.

SAMPLE #5: When I need a new outfit but am afraid you'll say it's too much money. Sometimes I'll get the outfit on my own, put it on my credit card and not tell you. I make myself feel angry that I can't talk with you about it and guilty that I'm keeping something from you.

***

Personal Example 1:

Personal Example 2:

Personal Example 3:

107

Front Door:

The direct approach involves knowing what you need or want and finding a way to express it clearly and respectfully to your spouse. It necessarily involves allowing yourself to be vulnerable, since vulnerability is an instant byproduct of sharing a need or want. For this reason, the front door approach requires more courage and trust than the side door. When your spouse responds to your front door approach with openness and acceptance, there is a wonderful opportunity for gratitude. When it is met with something else, there is an opportunity to clarify, negotiate and (as always) practice functional boundaries.

The front door approach represents a significant mental shift that replaces feelings of resentment with feelings of trust, safety and gratitude. When you start thinking, "Yes, we *can* get our needs met in this relationship," you are able to esteem your relationship and connect with your growing competencies as a couple. You may find that the front door is not as intimidating as it once seemed.

***

Look at the three examples you just listed for your side door approaches to needs and wants. *Can you find the front door?* What would it be like to honor your needs/wants by sharing them in a respectful and honest way with your spouse? As an example, read the following front door shift regarding side door Sample #2.

SAMPLE #2: *Front Door Approach*: "I would tell you that I had something I'd like to share with you and I would ask you if you were available to talk. Then I would tell you my challenge: It's really hard getting the kids ready for school in the morning and I would like to talk about ways to share some of the responsibilities. I would tell you that it's hard for me to ask because I'm a little bit scared of what your reaction might be, but that I'm trusting that I can share my needs with you and have it be OK. I would remind myself that my needs are valid, and that even a negative response from you does not make them any less so. I would also remind myself that we are equal, adult human beings, fully capable of negotiating a compromise when our needs or perspectives differ."

Personal Example 1: *Front Door Approach:*

108

Personal Example 2: *Front Door Approach:*

Personal Example 3: *Front Door Approach:*

Courageous Discovery Planned Intimate Experience:

What Can I Do?
(Bercaw & Bercaw)

Purpose and Goals:

One of the most important variables affecting couples recovery involves clarifying the automatic thoughts you have about yourself and your spouse. When you do, you are in a stronger position to change the thoughts you identify as being problematic. This cognitive restructuring is consistent with individual recovery principles around personal responsibility. For example, the Serenity Prayer supports us in knowing the difference between what we can and cannot change.

You will always be the sole owner of your thoughts. For this reason, the choice of examining them and changing them is yours and yours alone. If you are like everyone else, you will see how your own negative thoughts often wither in the face of reality. This PIE is designed to give you a chance to confront some of the "error messages" you may automatically send yourself. You will be challenged to "change the things I can" by replacing them with reality-based counterstatements, action steps and gratitude.

Instructions:

Please answer each of the following and share your responses with each other during your scheduled PIE time:

1. One negative or insecure thought I sometimes have about my marriage is:

2. When I allow myself to think rationally, I can identify the following reality-based, positive self-statements to counter the negative thought above:

      a.

      b.

3. One negative or insecure thought I sometimes have about my spouse is:

4. When I allow myself to think rationally, I can identify the following reality-based, positive self-statements to counter the negative thought above:

      a.

      b.

5. One negative or insecure thought I sometimes have about *myself* is:

6. When I allow myself to think rationally, I can identify the following reality-based, positive self-statements to counter the negative thought above:

      a.

      b.

7. Regarding my spouse, I am especially grateful for:

8. One thing I can do every day (or most days) to increase/maintain positive feelings for myself:

9. One thing I can do every day (or most days) to increase/maintain positive feelings toward my spouse:

11

Phase III: Revelation

Due to your hard work during the Courageous Discovery phase, you are in a good position to take more ownership of your healthy sexuality by knowing your bodies better. In the *Revelation* phase, you will learn about you and your spouse's sexual anatomy as well as your Sexual Response Cycles. The experiences in this phase provide a chance to feel positively connected to your genitals and to appreciate them as a valued part of your body with a healthy purpose and meaning. You will be asked to be specific about what you know about your body and how it typically responds. This can be a vulnerable experience and provides another opportunity to experience a deeper level of trust, intimacy and self-acceptance. It is not uncommon for spouses to endure years or decades of non-pleasurable sexual touch because they did not know what might feel better, or were too embarrassed to tell their partner what would feel better, or were afraid of the reaction they might get if they did tell. If you can relate in any way or suspect that your spouse might as well, then you are near putting those old ways behind. The old adage that "knowledge is power" is highly relevant: Many people realize that there was so much that they did not know about themselves or their spouse or both. Once you know, and once you share what you know, it becomes much easier to claim a healthy and functional sexuality and to enjoy the riches of sexual abundance with your spouse.

Mutual Agreements: Revelation
(Bercaw & Bercaw)

Instructions:

Read the following statements aloud and together and place your initials in the space next to each statement to show your agreement. If you are not sure that you agree, please circle the statement and remember to discuss it with your therapist at your next meeting.

1. We agree to pursue knowing our sexual selves (including our bodies) with openness and with respect for ourselves and each other. _____

2. As part of this openness, we agree to ask any questions we may have about the other's sexual thoughts, feelings and experiences. We also agree to remain open to being asked such questions. We commit to sharing our realities as authentically as we can. This applies also to the negative emotions that are easier to avoid than to acknowledge (fear, doubt, guilt, shame, anger, pain, etc). _____

3. We agree that despite any discomfort we may experience in our pursuit of greater awareness and understanding, the investment we are making in claiming a healthy and freely chosen sexuality will be worthwhile. _____

Revelation
Action Steps

• Know your body as an expert
• Know your spouse's body as an open-minded student
• Risk vulnerability through sharing/teaching about your body
• Consolidate specific gains

"Sexual Experience" Graph
(Bercaw & Bercaw)

Purpose and Goals:

This PIE is intended to help you learn and understand more about your sexual response pattern and to share this knowledge with your spouse. This is also the best way to learn and understand *your spouse's* sexual response pattern (far superior to reading about generic male/female sexual turn-ons in any magazine or book!). These experiences together will deepen your self-awareness of your body and mind as you choose to be sexual. As you identify *obstacles* in your sexual response, you can begin to understand how they evolved and how to address them. As you identify *erotic moments* in your sexual response, you may find opportunities for ongoing pleasure and can reveal more to your spouse about what those erotic moments are.

This deepening awareness and growing self-knowledge allows you to further embrace and claim your sexual self. You may realize that the old way of experiencing your sexuality was not *chosen* as much as it was *absorbed* from external sources. Now, as an adult *you* get to choose. The old way is being replaced with your freely chosen, intentional ways of thinking, feeling and being sexual. Being vulnerable through honestly sharing your new found sexual self in the presence of a safe and trusted partner builds intimacy in your coupleship.

Instructions:[24]

First, look at the differences in Sexual Response Cycle by gender (Appendix B). Note what is happening physically as each gender progresses through the various phases. Note instances where you have had a concern or difficulty with anything that you are reading about. Also note anything you may not have been aware of for yourself and for your spouse.

You are each going to make a graph of your sexual response. Take a blank piece of paper and fold into four equal columns (or draw vertical lines to create the same effect). Label the top of each column with a stage of the sexual response cycle (Excitement, Plateau, Orgasm, Resolution). Draw a line on your blank graph representing how your arousal progresses through the four stages of sexual response during a typical sexual experience. Draw your line upward to show increasing arousal and downward to show decreasing arousal. If you want your graph to reflect having an orgasm, your line should touch the upper edge of the paper under the orgasm phase. You may want to make several graphs to represent more than one sexual experience. For example, one graph could represent an intercourse experience when you reach orgasm and another could represent when you do not reach orgasm; for men, one could represent when you have difficulty with ejaculation, or another for when you cannot maintain an erection.

Be mindful of the times in your sexual experience where you experience either *obstacles* or *erotic moments* and plot those points at the appropriate places on your graph by using an "OB" or an "EM." Examples of obstacles are: Anxiety/nervousness;

114

pain; distractions (noise, thoughts, or images); fatigue; and of course, headaches! Erotic moments are highly individualized and often have little to do with orgasm. They are simply moments that we experience as highly charged with a strong element of arousal and excitement. Examples of erotic moments are: First skin to skin contact; removing underwear; deep and passionate kissing; slow, light kissing; eye contact during intercourse, caressing a spouse's breasts; the moment of penetration; having one's ear or finger or nipple "nibbled." The possibilities are endless.

When you share your graphs with each other, you are encouraged to use a *presentation format*: That is, give a presentation on your progression through the four stages of sexual response to your spouse. You will show your graph, and explain what is happening to you as you trace your line through the four stages on the graph (see sample transcript below). Do not be concerned that your spouse already knows this or that. There is much value in the process of actually discussing and presenting your sexual experience using the graph. When you are through, your spouse may ask questions or share thoughts and feelings about what you just shared. Then switch roles so your spouse can present while you listen.

Here is a sample transcript of one man's presentation:

"Let me walk you through my sexual response pattern during a typical intercourse experience. This is the very beginning of the Excitement Phase, where we have probably just sat down on the bed. I'm feeling a lot of things. I'm excited for what is about to happen, but I'm a little concerned about how things are going to go this time. We start kissing and holding each other and you can see on my graph I'm moving upward through the Excitement Phase. Then when you take your shirt or nightgown off, that's when I experience my first erotic moment – you see there's a little "EM" there on my graph. Then I move into the Plateau Phase as we keep kissing, and here's another erotic moment, when you first begin to touch my penis. But right after that is where I sometimes hit my first obstacle- there's the "OB" on my graph and you see how my graph line dips down a little bit. The obstacle is my insecurity about whether my erection is going to be okay or not. If I start feeding into the fear, then my arousal keeps dipping. But if I use the self-talk techniques I've learned and remember to look into your eyes as a way of maintaining my presence, I'm usually able to recover and go on to have a great time with you.

Here my line keeps going up through the Plateau Phase, and we're still enjoying foreplay. I've got another "EM" here- that's when I start touching your breasts and your vagina. It's a huge turn-on for me when we're touching each other at the same time. It seems like such a privilege! Then here in the Plateau Phase is about the time when you are guiding me into your vagina and we start having sex. Right after we start is where I have another obstacle- that's what this "OB" is for- it's when I sometimes wonder if you can tell that my erection might not be that great. But if I'm really turned on, I worry that I might not be able to last long enough for your orgasm to happen. So there you see my line dips a little, and sometimes, my erection never really comes back and, you know, those

115

are the times I end up feeling pretty much like a failure. I get really down on myself and our experience is over. So you see this line here goes all the way down.

But I made another graph to show what happens if I'm not focused on my erection and I'm not worried about ejaculating too soon. I'm able to linger in the Plateau Phase for a nice little while during sex and then I have my orgasm when I want to, which is usually right after you have yours. My arousal drops off quickly during the Resolution Phase, and that's when we usually get cleaned up and go to sleep."

Revelation Planned Intimate Experience:

Adult Show and Tell
(Bercaw & Bercaw)

Purpose & Goals:

In this PIE, you are going to be developing greater awareness and insight about the erotic parts of your body and presenting this information to your spouse. Thus, you will be reinforcing your intimacy: As you know yourself better, you can decide to share your knowledge with your spouse. You are able to choose to be open to your spouse's sharing also.

Because this experience is designed to be specific and detailed, some may feel awkwardness, fear or resistance. The first part of this PIE is the "Getting to Know Yourself" section. Many feel vulnerable with *themselves* as they explore their sexual and erotic areas. Therefore, inviting another person into this experience requires tremendous trust. There are two aspects of trust:

Trust in *oneself* ("I *can* handle this. My reward for tolerating any anxiety in this experience will be moving closer to claiming the healthy sexuality I always have deserved.") ("I can protect myself by practicing healthy boundaries when necessary; I can ask for what I need and set limits when necessary.")

Trust in one's *spouse* ("S/he is becoming a safer person to me based on our recent experiences and interactions. I am making a wise choice to trust him/her with my vulnerability").

In addition to these process goals, there is also a very practical element to this PIE: You are beginning to teach your spouse about what you know about your sexuality. No matter how much general knowledge one has about sexuality, there is a wide range of differences among people. Therefore, we want you to be as comfortable as possible while serving as your spouse's guide to your sexuality. This PIE is more clinical than any of the others. It aims to support you in becoming more comfortable using specific names for sexual anatomy. It is also an opportunity for each spouse to ask questions about the other's body and about the other's sexual experience.

Instructions for Part I:

In privacy, you will be examining your own genitals and will be using the anatomical sketches (at the end of Appendix B) to identify specific areas. Women may find it helpful to use a hand mirror to assist with an easier view. Take your time moving from the sketch to you own genitals, identifying each part as you go. Make mental notes along the way regarding what types of touch (if any) are most pleasurable for each of these parts. Also notice any feelings that may be triggered by this experience. It is not uncommon to have some negative emotions if you were raised with sex-negative messages, or if you have been abused or have had prior negative sexual experiences.

117

Instructions for Part II:

This part can occur in any room in which you can be comfortable and have privacy. The initiator (preferably the one who is *least* comfortable anticipating this PIE) is asked to set up the room in a way that feels honoring of the experience and promotes feelings of safety. For example, some feel more comfortable with soft candlelight or soothing background music.

As with the "Typical Sexual Response Graph" PIE, you are encouraged to approach this as a presentation to your spouse. The material you present is what you know about the sexual and erotic areas of your body. You will have the sketches of the male and female genitalia present and visible. Once both people are present and ready to begin, the person who is *most* comfortable with this PIE should be the first presenter. The presenter chooses a comfortable position, and using the sketches as a guide, begins identifying each specific part of his/her genitals to the listener (e.g. "This is my outer labia." "This is my clitoris." "This is my coronal ridge." "This is my urethral opening." "This is my frenulum."). It is helpful to use the clinical names for the parts for two reasons: first, to increase your comfort level with the parts of your bodies that many people are least comfortable with and second, to improve the accuracy of your sexual communication. You are more likely to know what the other is describing or asking for if you both use the same language. (Of course, you always have the option of substituting "pet" names for clinical names, just as long as you each know what the other means!)

The presenter also shares what it feels like when that specific part is touched and if any type of touch is preferred. For example: "This is my urethral opening but I do not like it touched directly." "This is my perineum and it feels good to have some steady pressure applied." As the presenter, you are encouraged to assume that your spouse *knows nothing* about your preferences. The listener is always free to ask questions of the presenter.

There should also be freedom for the presenter to *invite* the listener to *touch* the specific part being addressed or for the listener to ask permission to touch that part. For example, it is one thing to say, "I prefer a light, slow, indirect touch around my clitoris," or "I like it when you apply pressure to my perineum, but closer to my scrotum than to my anus," and quite another to show your spouse *exactly* what you mean. This hands-on experience is the best way to reinforce the verbal communication you give and receive. Remember that this is intended to be a clinical presentation and the demonstration is just that, an example. It should be clear, yet should take no longer than is necessary for the "lesson" to be understood.

As the presenter, you are also encouraged to address the areas of your body that are beyond your genitals, but that can be pleasurable when touched. For example, it might be that spot on your neck, ear, breast, forearm, buttocks, foot, calf or ankle that you know to be an erogenous zone *for you.*

After each of you has had a chance to present yourself to your spouse, there is a great opportunity to express gratitude to each other for the trust and commitment that was involved in the experience you just shared together. It is also time to reflect and write about the thoughts and feelings you were aware of while in the roles of presenter and listener. What was the best aspect of this PIE? Are you aware of anything that might have helped your experience be better? Do you think you might be more comfortable and/or knowledgeable about the sexual and erotic parts of your own and your spouse's body?

Planned Intimate Experience:

A "Hands-On" Lesson
(Bercaw & Bercaw)

Purpose & Goals:

This PIE is intended to help you take another step toward directly *teaching* your spouse about your touch preferences as well as *learning* about your spouse's preferences. Just as you recently were able to give and receive a "lesson" on the erotic and sexual areas of your bodies, you will expand this to include your entire bodies. You are continuing to develop self-awareness regarding your sensual/sexual preferences and conditions. As your self-awareness grows, you are taking ownership of *your* responsibility for *your* own pleasure. The basic premise is: *If you want your spouse to know what you like, you're going to need to show him/her!* Accepting this premise, you continue to clearly communicate your preferences. Allowing yourselves this vulnerability rewards you with a better understanding of each other's experiences. You are again being very proactive in taking steps to deepen the intimacy and trust in your relationship.

It is fundamental for each person to be as comfortable as possible while serving as their spouse's personal guide to their sensual and sexual preferences and conditions. While the teaching/learning component of this PIE may be similar to the "Adult Show and Tell," this PIE is less clinical. It is also an opportunity for each spouse to ask questions about the other's body and about the other's sexual experience.

Instructions:[25]

This PIE can occur in any room in which you can be comfortable and can have privacy. You will need enough space to lie next to each other and move around. The initiator is asked to set up the room in a way that feels honoring of the experience to come and in a way that promotes feelings of safety. For example, some people may feel more comfortable with soft candlelight or soothing background music. Enjoy a bath or shower together (no "Bikini Rule") as a warm-up before moving on to this PIE.

Each of you will have an opportunity to guide your spouse's hands all over and around your body. As the one doing the guiding, your job is to demonstrate clearly the type of touch that feels best to you. You are to take your spouse's hand with yours and move it all around your body. You may wish to either have your spouse's hand resting on top of yours or to have his/her hand under yours (skin to skin). Try to be as clear as you possibly can in your demonstrations: If you prefer a light, circular touch on your shoulders or a more firm up and down touch on the sole of your foot, now is the time to show your spouse exactly how to give that type of touch. It may be necessary to shift positions to allow access to most of your body.

As the one being guided, your goal is to be open to the lesson. This means that you will need to relax your hands and arms so your spouse can easily guide you. You may have questions as the lesson progresses and are encouraged to ask them. After the first lesson has been completed, in which you have slowly guided and have been guided around as much of the body as you can comfortably reach, it is time to switch roles.

While the lesson *includes* the breasts and genitals, it is intended to provide equal attention to all areas of the body. Since it includes the breasts and genitals, there is the potential for arousal. Whether arousal occurs or not is irrelevant: The focus remains on the process of sharing, teaching and learning that is so important for healthy intimacy and sexuality.

It is also important to keep in mind that even as you are trying to be clear in your lesson, there is likely to be some variability from one experience to the next: The same touch that feels wonderful on Sunday is not certain to have the same effect if repeated on Wednesday. In fact, it is that variability that contributes to the process of renewal and experimentation that can keep your sex lives interesting. You are not doing these lessons so you may become "perfect students." The goal is simply to develop a better understanding of some of your spouse's typical preferences while leaving plenty of room to be re-directed during future shared experiences.

***

After each of you has given your hands-on lesson, there is another opportunity to express gratitude to each other for the openness and trust involved in the experience you just shared. It is also time to reflect and write down the thoughts and feelings you had in each role. What was the best aspect of this PIE? Are you aware of anything that might have helped your experience be better? Do you have a better sense of how you and your spouse prefer to enjoy touch? Can you tell a difference between your comfort levels in discussing your preferences now versus when you first began the SRT program?

Revelation Planned Intimate Experience:

What I Know Now Part I
(Bercaw & Bercaw)

Purpose and Goals:

To allow each spouse to take a personal inventory about the specific areas of self-awareness and spousal-awareness that have been developed and/or enhanced. Being specific and concrete allows you to more clearly identify and claim the gains you made.

Instructions:

Please respond to the following as completely and specifically as possible. During your scheduled PIE time you will take turns reading your responses with the option of discussing any of them in more detail. (Examples from other SRT couples have been provided).

1. **What do you now know or understand about *yourself* that is more than you knew or understood before beginning the SRT program?**
   (e.g. "How easily I end up feeling resentful when I don't ask for what I need or want." "I feel small, like a child, when you ask me to do something." "I can keep commitments to myself and to my husband.")

2. **What do you now know or understand about your *spouse* that is more than you knew or understood before beginning the SRT program?**
   (e.g. "That you really love me despite all you know about me;" "How certain things are powerful triggers for you to feel scared and how your fear typically gets translated into anger;" "How unworthy and inadequate you have always felt and how you assume I see you that way too")

3. **What do you now know or understand about your *sexual* self that is more than you knew or understood before beginning the SRT program?**
(e.g. "I never realized that I can enjoy your touch just for the pleasure it brings and not have it be merely a stepping stone to sex;" "My sexual self is in the habit of just trying to get off. I'm seeing how much else there is to my sexuality and learning how to share it with you;" "When I am able to say up front that I am nervous it actually helps me release some of my anxiety- then I can enjoy whatever it is we are doing;" "I'm learning that I need to ask for what I want in order to get my pleasure, but I'm also realizing how hard it is for me to ask."

4. **What do you now know or understand about your spouse's sexual self that is more than you knew or understood before beginning the SRT program?**
(e.g. "You need to feel safe before you can enjoy our times together and I'm starting to understand what that means…;" "You can slow down and enjoy our shared moments instead of rushing ahead to your moment- and it's wonderful!")

12

Phase IV: Enhancement

The Enhancement phase is where things often begin to gel. By now, you are practiced in the discipline of being more present with each other. You also have made gains in your emotional intimacy by choosing to be more vulnerable with each other. Your increased presence and deepened emotional intimacy have allowed your sexual intimacy to grow. For these reasons, you probably have an enhanced sense of hope and optimism for your relationship. The Enhancement phase is about taking full advantage of your progress toward *functional sexual intimacy* and *sexual abundance*. The idea is that each of you will feel increasingly comfortable sharing your sexual realities with each other.

In this phase, you may notice more of an emphasis on *experimenting* with each other to see what feels comfortable and pleasurable, and then *teaching* each other what you've discovered. The exercises become more advanced, meaning breast and genital caressing is gradually being incorporated into the exercises. However, the focus is decidedly NOT on arousal, but rather on comfort, pleasure, and most definitely *fun!* If arousal does occur, (and the likelihood of it occurring increases as a function of the advanced nature of the experiences) that is a natural and positive part of the experience. Overall, the *Enhancement* phase is about capitalizing on the momentum you have gained by building on your increasing competencies. You are leading yourselves in the direction of the intimate relationship you envisioned earlier in this journey, growing closer and more confident with each step of the way.

Mutual Agreements: Enhancement

(Bercaw & Bercaw)

Instructions:

Read the following statements aloud together and place your initials in the space provided next to each one to indicate your agreement. (If you are not sure that you agree, please circle the statement so you remember to discuss it with your therapist at your next meeting).

1. We are grateful for our progress and are willing to continue making efforts to deepen our comfort and intimacy. _____

2. We appreciate each other's willingness to work toward our shared vision. _____

3. We embrace the novelty of experimenting with new types of touch with new experiences. _____

4. We will continue to risk being vulnerable as we share our sexual realities with each other. _____

Enhancement
Action Steps

• Enhance emotional intimacy and presence through touch and communication
• Enhance sexual intimacy as exercises become more advanced
• Develop Functional Sexuality through sharing sexual realities
• Welcome Sexual Abundance by sharing fun experiences

125

Enhancement Planned Intimate Experience:

Body Caressing (including breasts & genitals)
(Bercaw & Bercaw)

Purpose and Goals:
This PIE is a combination of the previous caressing PIEs, but without the "Bikini Rule." It capitalizes on the momentum you have gained by building on your increasing competencies. You are encouraged to continue experimenting with the new type of light, caressing touch you have been enjoying. You are encouraged to explore the sensual and pleasurable potential that various areas of your bodies offer. You are continuing to increase your capacity to slow things down and appreciate a broad range of sensual pleasure. Because of the work you have been doing, you now have the additional benefit of knowing your own touch preferences better, as well as those of your spouse. You likely are becoming more comfortable in sharing your preferences, and your intimacy is expanding accordingly.

Instructions:[26]
This experience is best suited for a room or area in your home where you can be comfortable lying down (bed, couch, blanket on floor). You will take turns caressing and being caressed over your entire bodies including (but not *focusing* on) the breasts and genitals. The breast and genitals are to receive as much attention as the elbows, calves, shoulders, face or any other area of the body. The initiator sets up the room in a way that feels honoring of the experience to come. Then, the initiator communicates that the room is set up and ready. Before beginning the caressing part of this PIE, enjoy some sensual bathing as a warm up to the caressing and also to promote feeling clean and fresh for this time together.

As the receiver, you are free to choose the amount of clothing you prefer while being caressed. You may choose to be completely naked, or may prefer to wear underwear, a t-shirt, or pajamas. There is no right or wrong attire for this exercise, as long as you both are comfortable. You each may choose to be in different states of undress. If you choose some light clothing, just know that eventually the goal will be to experience this PIE while both of you are naked.

Once both of you are in the room, the person who has agreed to be the first receiver finds a position that feels comfortable while lying face down, then communicates that s/he is ready. As the caresser, you are free to begin enjoying the experience of caressing the back of your spouse's body, from head to toe. Assume that your spouse is enjoying your touch unless s/he redirects you. As the receiver, you can be aware of any touch preferences you have and can share these preference with your spouse. As the caresser, you can remain open to any such feedback or redirection, understanding that such a communication is an act of intimacy in and of itself. Whenever the RECEIVER is ready to have the front of his/her body caressed, this should be stated. After a time of caressing both sides of the body, either of you may express when you feel ready to switch roles (receiver becomes caresser, caresser becomes receiver).

If either of you experiences anxiety that interferes with being present and engaged in the experience, it is your responsibility to communicate this. If this happens it may be wise to take a break, re-evaluate, and discuss how to proceed. Options include: Making adjustments to help the experience feel more comfortable or agreeing to stop the touching part of the experience and transition to recording the experience in your journals.

***

When each of you has had enough caressing, it is time to record your thoughts and feelings about this experience in your journals or in the space below. What did you enjoy the most? Would you choose to do this again, and if so, would you want to make any modifications? Did you encounter any barriers? What feelings were you aware of? How would you describe your comfort level? What are your feelings toward your spouse?

Note: Arousal may occur during this PIE because of the inclusion of breasts and genitals. If either spouse does become aroused, that is fine, but it is not the goal. It is important to surrender any *pursuit and/or monitoring of arousal* in order to allow yourselves to be optimally present with each other and to maintain optimal awareness of all that you are experiencing.

Enhancement Planned Intimate Experience:

Just a Kiss
(Bercaw & Bercaw)

Purpose and Goals:

This PIE provides a unique experience with a familiar activity. Some wonder, "Why is the kissing PIE so far back in the program after some of the more sexually involved things we've been doing together?" The answer is that kissing can be one of, if not *the* most intimate way of connecting with each other. The lips are one of the most sensitive areas on our entire bodies, and most of our sensory input comes from our heads; sight, smell, hearing, taste. When you bring together the most sensitive parts that allow you to experience the world, it is a true act of trust and intimacy. This may explain why some say they saw "fireworks" during a kiss!

Many people view kissing as a mere stepping stone to more overt sexual activities. The goal here is to emphasize the value of kissing as an *intimate experience of its own*. It is quite typical for couple's kissing to decline in frequency and enjoyment over time. It is also common for kissing to take on a signaling role, indicating that someone wants to have sex. There may be a gender correlation as well, namely that many wives really miss kissing their husbands. However, they hesitate to initiate kissing when they fear that it might miss-signal him that she also wants to be sexual. Now is the time for you to reclaim the pleasure of kissing.

This PIE provides another opportunity to identify your preferences and share them with your spouse. There is no right or wrong way to kiss because of the wide range of different preferences. The mutual openness to share and to learn continues to build trust and intimacy in your relationship.

Instructions:[27]

This experience can occur wherever you think would be most comfortable. You will be taking turns kissing and being kissed. The initiator sets up the room in a way that feels honoring of the experience to come. Then, the initiator communicates that the room is set up and ready.

Once both of you are in the room, decide who wants to be kissed first. That person finds a position that feels comfortable, and communicates to the one leading the kissing that s/he is ready. As the one *leading the kissing*, you are responsible for showing your spouse the kind of kissing you enjoy most. Consider kissing in areas other than the lips, such as the neck, ears, cheeks, or hair if this is something you enjoy. As you are leading in ways that *you* enjoy, remain open to your spouse's redirection. If you are not being redirected, you can safely assume that your spouse is enjoying your kissing.

As the person *being led* in the kissing, you can simply follow your spouse's lead, unless you are being led in a way that is not enjoyable or comfortable for you. If this occurs, then share your preference with your spouse. (e.g. "This is great, but could you keep going with less tongue?" or "I'm really enjoying this, but my neck is ticklish, could you please go back to kissing my lips?") When you have had enough time, switch roles so that you each get a turn leading.

The spirit of this PIE is fun, open, and experimenting! Don't be afraid to laugh, and try kissing in some new ways, or to remember how much fun you had with kissing earlier in your relationship.

***

When you both have had enough time kissing, it is time to record your thoughts and feelings about this experience in your journals. (What did you enjoy the most? What did you learn about how your spouse prefers kissing? Did you encounter any barriers? What feelings were you aware of? Would you like to do more kissing in the future? How would you describe your comfort level? What are your feelings toward your spouse?)

Note: This experience is not designed to include any touching of breasts and/or genitals. Also, if either spouse does become aroused that is fine, but it is not the goal. It is important to surrender any *pursuit and/or monitoring of arousal* in order to allow yourselves to be optimally present with each other and to maintain optimal awareness of all that you are experiencing.

Note: Some people never have been comfortable with kissing. If this is the case for either one of you, discuss what your obstacles have been in the past and how you might modify the experience to work around this sensitivity (e.g. agree to try closed-mouth only kissing the first time; try kissing each other's hands as a bridge to kissing on the lips and face).

Enhancement Planned Intimate Experience:

Surprise Me!
(Bercaw & Bercaw)

Purpose and Goals:

This PIE is designed to help you answer the question, *"Are we having fun yet?"* Fun and joy go hand in hand, leading us into moments of spiritual connection. Recovery, including this program, does not always have to be so serious! We know how important it is to "keep it light" in the bedroom. Hopefully, this PIE provides a fun, new way to continue expanding your range of sensual and sexual pleasure. Be open to laughter and playfulness into your bedroom. Welcome the light moments. Embrace what you cannot predict or change. Let go of sexual perfectionism. Have fun with this!

Instructions:[28]

This experience can occur wherever you think would be most comfortable lying down. You will be taking turns caressing and being caressed. The initiator sets up the room in a way that feels honoring of the experience to come. Then the initiator communicates that the room is set up and ready. As with previous caressing PIEs, enjoy a shower or bath together before beginning.

You are each asked to bring three objects to the room. The criteria for selecting these objects is simply that you think your spouse might enjoy the sensation of being caressed with each object. Do not let each other know what the objects are just yet!

Once both of you are ready, decide who will be caressed first. That person then lies naked (or with the minimum amount of clothing that feels comfortable) and face down with his/her back exposed. As the caresser, use each object to stroke your spouse's back for a period of time that is adequate to give your spouse a sense of how each object feels. It can be fun to have the receiver try to guess the identity of each object.

As the receiver, once you have had a chance to experience the sensations of each object, you are asked to choose the one object that you would prefer to be caressed with *all over your body*. The caresser uses that object to caress both sides of the receiver's body, from head to toe. When the receiver has enough time being caressed, it is time to switch roles and the same process is repeated. Remember to keep redirecting each other as necessary in order to really get the most out of this PIE.

When you both have had enough time, record your thoughts and feelings about this experience in your journals. (What did you enjoy the most? What did you learn about your comfort with spontaneity and creativity? Did you encounter any barriers? What feelings were you aware of? Would you like to do more of this in the future?)

Enhancement Planned Intimate Experience:

Bedroom Soccer & Mutual Genital Caress
(Bercaw & Bercaw)

Purpose and Goals:

This PIE (Planned Intimate Experience) is designed to help you to continue to keep things light in the bedroom as you experiment with new ways of enjoying each other. *Bedroom Soccer* is intended to be pure fun, even silly. The PIE is designed so you can flow right from Bedroom Soccer into the *Mutual Genital Caress*. Taken together, these activities consolidate many of the experiences you have had in previous PIEs.

Instructions:[29]

This experience can occur wherever you think would be most comfortable. The initiator sets up the room in a way that feels honoring of the experience to come. Then, the initiator communicates that the room is set up and ready. Before beginning this PIE, again enjoy a bath or shower together (remembering the guidelines of the Sensual Bathing PIE). When you have finished bathing or showering you are ready to begin.

Decide who will be caressed first, and then that person then lies naked with his/her back exposed. As the caresser, you can use any part of your body to caress your spouse's body EXCEPT your hands (just like soccer - no hands allowed!). Feel free to experiment by using parts of your body you would not normally use (your hair, cheeks, lips, arms, feet, chest, nose, tongue and even your breasts and genitals). The receiver can turn over to enjoy pleasuring on the front of his/her body. Be as creative as you like, as long as your spouse is comfortable with what you are doing.

After each of you has had a chance in each role, it is time to move into the second part of this PIE. Lying closely together and facing each other, breathe deeply and look into each other's eyes for as long as you like. Then enjoy a time of mutual caressing and kissing (*the "No Hands" rule is no longer in effect*). You are free to enjoy caressing your spouse's genitals and having your own caressed at the same time. Remember to keep using the process of redirecting and teaching each other, so you are asking for the type of touch you want and showing your spouse how it's done. Continue kissing and caressing until one or both of you would like to conclude your experience. Given the erotic touching involved, you may choose to follow your arousal to the point of orgasm. If this is the case, enjoy it as part of your experience, but do not make it a goal for the experience.

***

It is time to record your thoughts and feelings about this experience in your journals. (What did you enjoy the most? How did you like the no-hands rule? How did the simultaneous pleasuring feel different from the individual caressing you had been practicing? Did you encounter any barriers? What feelings were you aware of? Would you like to do more of any of this PIE in the future?)

<u>NOTE</u>: Sometimes the topic of oral sex comes up during the "No Hands" part. If so, it may present an opportunity to discuss how you each feel about oral sex. Remember to allow for plenty of room for different feelings and preferences. There is no "right or wrong" way to feel about this. The important thing is to be as clear as you can in expressing your preferences and comfort level as you remain open to hearing your spouse's as well.

For example, a couple might involve a man who enjoys receiving oral sex, but might not be comfortable pleasuring his wife orally. This might be a source of frustration or concern for her. In this example, it can be helpful as well as intimacy enhancing, for the couple to explore what it is about pleasuring his wife's genitals that has not felt comfortable. This could lead to a discussion about what could be done to help the husband feel more comfortable with this type of pleasuring. For example, if the husband's discomfort is rooted in his insecurity ("I don't know what I'm doing down there."), his wife might be open to giving him a tutorial. If his discomfort is rooted in a hygiene concern, it might help to experiment with oral pleasuring immediately after bathing or showering. Whatever it is, the most important thing is to be able to discuss it openly.

Enhancement Planned Intimate Experience:

"Pick-A-PIE"
(Bercaw & Bercaw)

Purpose and Goals:
  This PIE (Planned Intimate Experience) is a model for embracing spontaneity by connecting with what you prefer in the moment. It takes advantage of the now expanded menus for sensual and sexual pleasure you have developed through the SRT Program. What you will find in this PIE is that *everything* is on the menu. All you need to do is know what you want to order! You will still maintain some structure, just as in the previous PIEs but now you get to decide what to do based on whatever you prefer in the moment.

Instructions:
  This experience can occur wherever you think would be most comfortable. You will be taking turns pleasuring each other. The initiator sets up the room in a way that feels honoring of the experience to come. Then, the initiator communicates that the room is set up and ready.
  Once you are both in the room, decide who will be the first receiver. As the receiver, you request the type of pleasuring that you would like. It can be *anything* that you have done already in the SRT program. For example, you might say, "I'd like some total body caressing with a shower first and no Bikini Rule." As the spouse hearing this request, you can consider whether your spouse's request is something you can agree to. If so, you are free to proceed with the activity. If not, you can communicate to your spouse that you are not comfortable with that specific request at this specific time. You might wish to suggest another activity or ask if there is a second option your spouse might prefer. Remember that it is OK to have different feelings about being sensual and sexual at any given time and that it is important to communicate so you can negotiate.
  Switch roles after the first round of giving and receiving pleasure and repeat the same process as above. Then it is once again time to record your thoughts and feelings about this experience in your journals. (What did you enjoy the most? How did you experience the process of asking for what you wanted? How about the experience of being asked? Did you encounter any barriers? What feelings were you aware of? Would you like to set up more times like this in the future?)

13

Phase V: Integration

Entering this fifth and final phase of SRT, you have likely made significant changes in how you think about sexuality as individuals and as a couple. You may be more aware than ever of the contrast between your former ways of interacting and your new, intimacy-centered way of interacting. These shifts are beginning to feel more real, more stable and easier to trust. When you experience roadblocks (as everyone does), now you can rely on what you've learned, confident that you will be able to work through challenges as *partners*, with room for both of your realities and a spirit of mutual respect.

The Integration phase is about recognizing how far you've come and claiming all of the victories you have achieved. But it is also a time to acknowledge that there is more to be done and always will be. It is important to bear in mind that perfect harmony is not the end goal of the journey you are on. Rather than perfection and the absence of conflict, we are aiming for consistently different ways of thinking, feeling and relating. Those goals are realistic, manageable and renewable.

Mutual Agreements: *Integration*
(Bercaw & Bercaw)

Instructions:

Read the following statements aloud together and place your initials in the space provided next to each one to indicate your agreement. (If you are not sure that you agree, please circle the statement so you remember to discuss it with your therapist at your next meeting).

1. We have deep gratitude for each other's partnership and commitment through this challenging process of healing. _____

2. We commit to thoroughly examine the journey we've been on   together during the course of this program so we may identify the specific gains we have made.

_____

3. We value the need to create a specific plan in order to maximize the potential for these gains to be maintained and further enjoyed. _____

4. We commit to regularly review our plan. _____

5. We are open to modifying our plan as we continue to experiment, experience and evolve. _____

Integration
Action Steps

- Consolidate areas of growth and identify ongoing growth areas
- Create shared vision of healthy sexual intimacy
- Create plan to make your vision realistic by integrating SRT concepts into your coupleship
- Commit to regularly review your plan with each other and with therapist (as necessary)

Integration Planned Intimate Experience:

My Spiritual Moment
(Bercaw & Bercaw)

Purpose and Goals:

As you come down the homestretch of the SRT process, one of the things you may be aware of is the level of connection you feel with each other, and how it feels different from the past. As you look back on the many experiences you have shared with each other during this process, one or more may stand out for you as especially meaningful moments of connection. You might even go so far as to place moments like these in the "spiritual" category. It might not be the first time you have ever felt this way in your spouse's presence, but by now you may have a better idea about the conditions that need to be present in order to achieve this level of connection. You know that having a spiritual connection with your spouse is not happenstance. It is a destination reached with each other that results from being present. You can surrender to those moments and be closely connected with your reality.

The authenticity and vulnerability that characterizes these shared moments often lead to very powerful emotions and sensations (gratitude, joy, love, passion, pleasure, etc). By reflecting on these moments personally and sharing them with your spouse, you not only reinforce the growing and strengthening bond between you, but you give rise to the hope that you can continue to nurture your spiritual connection in the future.

Instructions:

Reflect on a time during the SRT process that you experienced a spiritual moment in your spouse's presence, and write about it as it unfolded chronologically. As you write, be mindful of the following:

- Was there any *relevant context* for this moment? (e.g. the first time you had been naked together in over a year; a recent loss; a recent accomplishment)
- What was actually *happening* at the time?
- What *emotional feelings* were you aware of?
- What *bodily sensations* were you aware of?
- Why does this moment stand out?
- What made it feel spiritual?

Share your writing with each other during your PIE time.

Integration Planned Intimate Experience:

Putting It All Together
(Bercaw & Bercaw)

Purpose and Goals:

This PIE (Planned Intimate Experience) is the next natural step in your progression of caressing PIEs. Each of you has been pursuing a process of significant change. It is founded on the belief that you deserve to discover and nurture your healthy sexual selves in the context of increasing healthy intimacy with each other. Now you have an opportunity to draw from the broader menu of sensual pleasures you have developed with each other, and to add another item. While this PIE includes having intercourse, you are encouraged to maintain a perspective that rather than the "main course" this is merely the "next course." This is a time to celebrate your privilege to be able to enjoy each other in this special way.

Instructions:

This experience can occur wherever you think would be most comfortable. The initiator sets up the room in a way that feels honoring of the experience to come. Then, the initiator communicates that the room is set up and ready. Before beginning this PIE, be sure to enjoy a bath or shower together. When you have finished bathing or showering you are ready to begin.

Once both of you are ready, decide who will be caressed first. Take turns caressing each other's bodies as you have done many times before in the SRT program. You also may choose to enjoy a time of mutual caressing. You may kiss passionately and to continue to experiment with the types of touch you now know that you and your spouse enjoy. After you have spent some time enjoying each other in various ways, communicate when you are ready to move into position for intercourse.

Agree to the position that you think would be a comfortable way to start. Take some time to enjoy genital to genital stimulation without entry. You may wish to use a personal lubricant to enhance your comfort and pleasure.

After you have enjoyed external genital to genital pleasuring and want to move toward intercourse, verbally communicate this to your spouse. It is important to move slowly and in concert with one another. Since it is the woman's body that is being entered, it is important that she be the one controlling the timing and pace of entry, as well as guiding the penis into the vagina. After entry has occurred, you may wish to enjoy some "quiet vagina," time, where you rest quietly together. If both of you are comfortable at this point, proceed to moving slowly with gentle thrusting. Continue to communicate about your comfort and preferences, redirecting each other as needed (including switching positions).

You may wish to follow your arousal to the point of orgasm, although that is not the *goal* for the time together. After you have concluded your intercourse time, and after taking any necessary time to clean up, you can hold each other in your arms (think: "Quiet Cuddle"). Maintain your presence with each other in this way until you are ready to bring this PIE to a close.

***

Although you may be in a state of relaxation, it is time to record your thoughts and feelings about this experience in your journals. (What did you enjoy the most? Did you encounter any barriers? What felt different/similar compared to your previous intercourse experiences with each other? What feelings were you aware of?) What are you feeling now?)

NOTE: You may notice a tendency toward your old intercourse patterns, whatever they may have been. Consider that you now have an opportunity to decide which of them to keep in the mix, which ones you'd like to discard and any new ideas you might want to try. For example, the couple that for years has had a predictable pattern of: [Kissing→ genital stimulation→ her orgasm→entry → his orgasm → done] may want to experiment with a longer period of kissing, or to linger longer after intercourse, and to approach their intercourse as more than being primarily for him to reach orgasm.

Integration: Planned Intimate Experience

Shall We Dance?
(Bercaw & Bercaw)

Purpose and Goals:

This activity combines passion, fun and eroticism with music and dancing. If you do not consider yourself a good dancer, do not worry- no real skill is required, just an openness to letting loose a little bit. This PIE is a great example of how your SRT efforts have really paid off. Now more than ever you can freely enjoy each other in ways that you might not have imagined in the past. Many people find music to be a spiritual gateway. Even if that has not been your experience, the idea is to be open to whatever moves you during this PIE. Let the music play!

Instructions:

You will need a device that plays your favorite songs (iPod, CD Player, etc.). Each of you will come prepared with two songs that you would like to dance to with your spouse. There is no expectation regarding what type of music you choose. You can choose from a full range of genres and tempos, the only criteria being that you think it would be a fun song for this PIE.

After bathing or showering, get back into some light, comfortable clothing. Then, decide who will play the first song. Dance to this song with your clothes on. When this song is over, it is the other person's turn to play a song. As the music begins, each of you will remove the other's outer clothes, leaving only your undergarments on for this dance. When this song is over, the musical choice swings back to the person who played the first song. You will each remove the other's undergarments so you can dance naked to this song.

When this third song is over, it is time to alternate musical choice again. You might want to keep dancing where you have danced the previous three songs, or you might wish to get into bed and enjoy each other there as the music plays on. There is no predetermined end point for this PIE. If it leads to sexual touching or intercourse, great! If not, then at least you have found a new dance hall right in your own home!

***

After you have had enough fun with this PIE, it is time to record your thoughts and feelings about this experience in your journals. What did you enjoy the most? Did you encounter any barriers? What feelings were you aware of? What are you feeling now? Is this an experience you would want to try again?

139

Integration Planned Intimate Experience:

Gratitude Letter
(Bercaw & Bercaw)

Purpose and Goals:
Gratitude is one feeling that is universally experienced in recovery. It is likely that you have vastly enhanced awareness of your gratitude for many things resulting from the work you have done in recovery. Because you have been working so closely with each other throughout the SRT program, you are probably aware of feelings of gratitude for what you have achieved and what you have appreciated about each other. Now is a time to connect with those feelings and to share them with each other.

One of the most powerful ways to increase intimacy is to feel grateful for another person and to express your gratitude directly. When we allow ourselves to *experience* gratitude, we open ourselves to move in the direction of the person that we feel grateful. This requires some vulnerability. When we actually *express* gratitude, we embrace the additional layer of vulnerability that is involved.

Instructions:
Now is a time to connect with those feelings and to share them with each other. Start by making a list of as many things that you can think of that you appreciate regarding your spouse's participation in and contributions to your SRT program. You may find the following questions helpful in organizing your thoughts:

- Recall when you signed the SRT Commitment Contract; what was your biggest concern and what did you most want your spouse to be aware of?
- When were you aware that your spouse was doing something that did not come naturally and therefore required some additional thought or focus or courage?
- When do you recall your spouse being sensitive or aware of your feelings during a difficult time for you?
- When were you aware of your spouse following through on a commitment?

Once you complete your list, write a letter to your spouse expressing your gratitude for each item on your list. Take turns reading your letters to each other during your scheduled PIE time, and make a copy for your spouse to keep. Finally, share your reactions to hearing each other's letter as well as the process you took to prepare the letter you wrote. Remember that the feelings of gratitude you connected with during this PIE were there *before* this PIE, just waiting to be embraced, enjoyed and shared.

Integration Planned Intimate Experience:

What I Know Now: Part II
(Bercaw & Bercaw)

Purpose and Goals:
 This communication PIE allows each of you to take a personal inventory regarding the specific areas of awareness that have been developed or enhanced. Being specific and concrete allows you to more clearly identify and claim the gains you have made. Your answers to this questionnaire, combined with those from Part I in the Revelation Phase, will form the basis for your *Lifetime Blueprint for Functional Sexual Intimacy.* Here is another opportunity for gratitude, as you are aware of knowing so much more now than you did "back then."

Instructions:
 Please review the responses you had to the following four questions from Part I of this PIE back in the Revelation Phase. The questions are reprinted below so you can make any additions that have arisen from your recent experiences. During your scheduled PIE time you will take turns reading your responses with the option of discussing any of them in more detail. (Examples from other SRT couples have been provided).

1. **What do you know or understand about *yourself* now that is more than you knew or understood before beginning the SRT program?**

   (e.g. "How easily I end up feeling resentful when I don't ask for what I need or want." "That I feel very small, like a child, when you ask me to do something." "I can keep commitments to myself and to my husband.")

2. **What do you know or understand about your *spouse* now that is more than you knew or understood before beginning the SRT program?**

   (e.g. "That you really love me despite all you know about me;" "How certain things are powerful triggers for you to feel scared and how your fear typically gets translated into anger." "How unworthy and inadequate you have always felt and how you assume I see you that way, too.")

141

3. **What do you know or understand about your *sexual* self now that is more than you knew or understood before beginning the SRT program?**

(e.g. "I never realized that I can enjoy your touch just for the pleasure it brings and not have it be just a stepping stone to sex;" "My sexual self is in the habit of just trying to get off. I'm seeing how much else there is to my sexuality and learning how to share it with you;" "When I am able to say up front that I am nervous it actually helps me release some of my anxiety. Then I can enjoy whatever it is we are doing;" "I'm learning that I need to ask for what I want in order to get my pleasure, but I'm also realizing how hard it is for me to ask." "How that little bit of fear is still there when I think about sharing my sexual reality." "That I usually enjoy myself sexually once I get into an experience, even if I don't start the experience with much, if any, desire.")

4. **What do you know or understand about your spouse's sexual self now that is more than you knew or understood before beginning the SRT program?**

(e.g. "You need to feel safe before you can enjoy our times together and I'm starting to understand what that means...;" "You can slow down and enjoy our shared moments instead of rushing ahead to your moment- and it's wonderful!")

142

Finishing Instructions:

In the next PIE, you are going to create a Master List of everything you have come to value through your SRT experiences. But first you must create your own individual lists. The following steps and the boxes on the next page will guide you.

    a. Look back at all of your responses from the *What I Know Now PIEs*. Make a list of the themes that stand out as being especially helpful or important to you. For example, you might notice themes around safety, scheduling, slowing down, prioritizing, presence, pleasure, fun, redirection, spirituality, etc.

    b. Respond to the questions below. They will help you connect with additional principles you have come to value. Make additions to the list above as you become aware of these connections.

- **What leads to positive sexual experiences for you?**
- **What have you found helpful in identifying and sharing your sexual realities?**
- **What obstacles have you encountered in this process?**
- **What have you found helpful in working around these obstacles?**
- **What are meaningful ways of nurturing the "living room" of your relationship?**
- **In what ways have you experienced *Sexual Abundance?***

List of important themes, concepts, and principles from the *WHAT I KNOW NOW* PIEs:

_____
_____
_____
_____
_____
_____
_____
_____
_____

List other themes, concepts and principles from questions on previous page:

_____
_____
_____
_____
_____
_____
_____
_____

Now *rank each item* on your lists above by placing a number next to it.

Finally, bring these lists to your next PIE, *"Lifetime Blueprint for Functional Sexual Intimacy and Abundance."*

Integration: Planned Intimate Experience:

Lifetime Blueprint for Functional Sexuality Intimacy and Abundance
(Bercaw & Bercaw)

Purpose and Goals:
     You have invested much in this process to create a new relationship grounded in intimacy. Now it is time to develop a master plan to make sure you can enjoy and build upon what you have created in an ongoing and practical way. Your Lifetime Blueprint will be a written record of everything you have come to value in your progress to date. It is not only a list of these values, but also an *action plan*. Detailing the proactive steps required to continue your progress makes any short or long term goals much more realistic. It also helps to insure that you continue living in accordance with your values. When you see your Lifetime Blueprint, you may rightly conclude that *you have made something out of nothing.* Without your courage, fortitude and mutual commitments to this process you would be back where you started.

Instructions:
Part I: Compare the lists each of you made at the end of your last PIE (*"What I Know Now II"*) Notice items that are similar and any items that are only on one of your lists. Once you have compared your lists, *merge them into one Master List*, and rank the items in order with the most important items near the top. The general rule is, "If it is important to *one* of us, it should be on our Master List." Some negotiation may be required. For example, let's say your spouse's list includes, "Scheduling time to enjoy each other," and yours does not. Then it would be helpful to reach a compromise regarding where scheduling could fit on your Master List.

_____
_____
_____
_____
_____
_____
_____
_____
_____
_____
_____
_____
_____
_____
_____
_____
_____
_____
_____
_____
_____
_____

Part II: For each item on the Master List, you will need to write a clear action statement regarding how you can live in accordance with that value. For example, if the value "Scheduling time to enjoy each other," makes it onto your Master List, an appropriate action statement would be, "We will meet each Sunday after putting the kids to bed to agree on at least one scheduled time during the week to enjoy a time of sensual/sexual intimacy."

The series of clear action statements, taken together, become a blueprint for you to follow for the rest of your lives. Like any good plan, it is designed to produce desired outcomes when followed consistently, yet flexible enough to be adjusted from time to time. Above all else, it is uniquely yours. Your experiences during SRT were yours, the values that grew out of those experiences are yours and the action steps in your Lifetime Blueprint are yours.

It may be helpful to refer to the sample on the following page as you convert your Master List into the Lifetime Blueprint itself. When you have finished with your Lifetime Blueprint, you have crossed the finish line of the SRT program. In Chapter 14, we conclude with thoughts on your reaching this milestone in your couple's recovery.

Lifetime Blueprint for Functional Sexual Intimacy and Abundance
(sample)

1. We will coordinate our scheduled PIE time for the next week each Sunday at 8PM.
2. We will meet for RCI's on the 1st and 3rd Sundays of the month at 8:15PM (following PIE scheduling) (Jack initiates).
3. We will meet for Daily Shares every night at 8:30 (except Wed- group night- 9PM)(alternate responsibility for initiating on weekly basis.)
4. We will reserve two PIEs/week for pleasuring that leads to intercourse and one PIE that does not.
5. We will define successful experiences by how present and connected we feel (not by how intense the experience is).
6. We will kiss passionately on a regular basis, just for the sake of kissing (not just during our sexual times).
7. We commit to practicing the Guidelines for Communicating (Appendix A) as a general rule, but especially when we feel uncomfortable or anxious or we want or need something. This works for us!
8. We are each responsible for our own pleasure: We will redirect and welcome redirection in keeping with this approach.
9. We will take one weekend per quarter for our marriage (go to a B&B; camping trip; hotel on the beach).
10. We will each continue to work our recovery programs.
11. We will review our Lifetime Blueprint at our 1st Daily Share of the month and ask: "How are we doing?" (Then use Guidelines for Communicating!)
12. We will meet with our therapist on a quarterly basis to review and revise our Lifetime Blueprint.

_____   _____
Jack   Rebecca

14

A New Day Dawns

If you are reading this chapter, you have accomplished a great deal in reaching the finish line of the SRT program and deserve congratulations. Like most great accomplishments in life, it is only reached with courage and dedication. We envisioned this destination when we were developing the logo for our website. We chose an image of the sun rising on a new day, which symbolizes our treatment philosophy. It represents one of the most basic elements of our human existence: With each new day, a new beginning, and all of the hope that comes with it. In reaching the conclusion of the SRT program, you have established a new framework for a lifetime of well-founded hopefulness.

In the beginning of this book, you were offered hope in the form of the SRT program, a vehicle to get you to where you wanted to be in your relationship. Through SRT, we tried especially to help you heal the part of your relationship that had been most obviously affected by the addiction, your sexual intimacy. We asked you to understand that any sexual healing would need to rest upon a solid foundation of emotional intimacy.

You have been working in a mutually committed way on both of these tracks. Because of your efforts, you now know yourselves and each other better than ever before. You feel more comfortable sharing your realities with each other honestly and respectfully. You have become more skilled in moving toward each other while maintaining your individuality. Your emotional intimacy is noticeably improved, because there is a much more secure attachment bond between you than ever existed before.

The process of sharing yourselves in this way has followed you right into your bedroom, where you now enjoy a greater sense of freedom, presence, joy and fun. You realize how your sexual selves have evolved during this process and how the sexual intimacy you share has been enhanced. By choosing to practice *Functional Sexual Intimacy,* your menu of pleasurable activities has been expanded, and your comfort level has grown. You are enjoying the positive flow of the *Circulation Model* and are connecting with the essence of *Sexual Abundance*: a renewable system of intimacy and pleasure that seems to just keep getting better.

These positive trends are not due to coincidence but to your own actions. You are feeling more comfortable in nurturing the sexual intimacy in your marriage and allowing yourself to be nurtured by it. As a result, you feel more trusting of the gains you have made, knowing that you have the power to keep being proactive. As you look back on your SRT experiences, you can see how your times together have become more playful, fun and experimental. What once was characterized by fear or resentment is now characterized by trust and openness. You have worked diligently to make this wonderfully transformative shift and many others. As a result, you are aware of what you now have in place and of what great potential the future holds. Now you can *keep* reaping the benefits of the work you have done.

Nevertheless, you should allow for those times or cycles when one of you is less available than you would prefer. You can understand and even expect that each of you, by virtue of your humanity, will sometimes lapse back into pre-SRT ways of thinking, feeling and behaving. When you slip back into old, dysfunctional ways of relating, you now are resilient enough to pull yourselves back into the new, functional ways to which you have committed. These occasional slips feel different now than pre-SRT because *you can talk about them.* When you do talk about them, you know how to do so safely, without blame or shame. You understand that your greatest victories as a couple are not defined by the absence of difficulties, but by your resilience in response to them

We take for granted that the sun will rise tomorrow. But we do not take for granted that we can rest on our relationship laurels. That is why you developed your *Lifetime Blueprint.* It represents the most important concepts you have learned and the best practices you have developed. What happens from here on out is fairly predictable: If you consistently review and follow your Blueprint, you will consistently experience a deepening of your sexual and emotional intimacy. Just like you may have heard before, *"It works if you work it!"*

So, it is all there for you now: A new, intimacy-based system that you can enjoy and continue developing for the rest of your lives. This ongoing commitment to intimacy keeps the sun rising in your relationship, warming your hearts, and shining brightly on the new, precious jewel that is your marriage. You have taken your relationship's weaknesses and transformed them into great strengths. Now, with your shared commitment to recovery through SRT, you may find yourselves wondering, "How *GOOD* can this get?" May this question occur to you often and may you always seek its answer in truth and love.

Practicing Functional Boundaries [12]
(to be read together after signing the Couple's Commitment Contract)

Practicing functional boundaries is a very personal thing. It is first and foremost an act of self-respect, but it also allows us to respect others with whom we are relating. When we practice functional boundaries we are being protective of ourselves without being overprotective. Thus, we must find ourselves *worthy* of protecting in the first place. Only then we will not allow ourselves to be victims. We are also containing ourselves without being too self-censoring. That is how we can share whatever is true for us without being offensive in the process.

As we protect and contain ourselves in our relationships, we are able to more clearly identify what is true for us at any given time. This way of living opens allows us to experience *functional intimacy: When we are able to share our truth and receive the truth of another without being either too vulnerable or invulnerable.* If we are too vulnerable, it can feel as if another person's reality is or should be our reality. On the opposite extreme, if we are "walled off" it will not be possible to experience any meaningful intimacy.

Boundaries involve two systems, the *external boundary* and the *internal boundary*. The external boundary protects and contains the body and is used in physical and sexual intimacy. The internal boundary protects and contains the mind and emotions and is used during emotional intimacy.

External Boundary System: An example of how the external boundary system works for you is when you want to kiss your spouse, and you would ask him/her, "Can I kiss you?" Similarly, if your spouse is moving toward you with some physical affection, you might think to yourself, "Is this what I want right now?" If the answer is "yes" you would enjoy the affection, but if the answer is no, you would respectfully decline your spouse's advance or invitation.

Internal Boundary System: The internal boundary system has two components, the *Talking Boundaries* and the *Listening Boundaries*. The following principles are very important to keep in mind when using the talking and listening boundaries:

Internal Talking Boundary: The spirit of the Talking Boundary is simple: You are respectfully sharing your reality *in order to be known.* You have the option of sharing a thought and/or feeling and you might have a request that relates to the thought or feeling you share. You are mindful that you are not sharing your reality in order to convince your spouse that yours is the "right" or "correct" perspective. You are not trying to manipulate or control your spouse's reality. You let go of the outcome as you engage in

---

[12] This model of Functional Boundaries is used with permission from Pia Mellody, who developed the concepts and taught them to us. We have made certain adaptations, but the key components of this entire section are hers.

a real act of intimacy: simply stating what is true for you. You do not blame anyone for the emotions you are feeling. They are your emotions and you own them.

<u>Internal Listening Boundary</u>: The spirit of the Listening Boundary is also straightforward: You are respectfully listening *so that you may know your spouse better*. You are mindful that you are not listening so that you can respond defensively. You recognize that your spouse's reality need not become your reality. You try to appreciate that your spouse is engaging in an act of intimacy by sharing his/her truth with you, even if it is very different from your perspective. You remind yourself that you are not responsible for your spouse's emotions.

When both of you are consistently practicing functional boundaries, there is *plenty of room* for two separate people (from two different backgrounds, with two different life experiences, two different educations and even two different bodies) to see things quite differently if they spend enough time together. Rather than living in fear of sharing your reality or receiving your spouse's reality, these boundary systems allow you to speak from your truth and to what is true for your spouse. This model allows you to experience connection while maintaining your individuality.

You might notice how awkward it feels to begin practicing this new approach to interacting with each other. While it is true that it may not be "natural" to interact this way, it is also often true that what comes naturally does not serve us very well. If you stick with this new approach despite it feeling artificial, mechanical or unnatural, you will be rewarded with a significantly enhanced ability to have real conversations about things that matter to you.

Guidelines for Communicating: The communication system outlined below has been designed to bring the principles detailed above down to a practical level. You begin with a request, end with a request, and have three shares in the middle.

<u>Speaker:</u> Your primary goal is to let your spouse know what your reality is in a respectful way.

1. **REQUEST** time: "There is something I'd like to share with you- is now a good time?" If the answer is "yes" proceed to #2. If the answer is no, ask, "When do you think might be a better time?"
2. **SHARE** what happened: Set it up- what did you hear or see or experience that you'd like to share? (e.g. "When we were talking at the table you got up and left the room without saying anything and you had a look on your face."
3. **SHARE** your thoughts about what happened: What meaning did you give to what happened? (e.g. "What I made up in my mind about that is you were upset with me for some reason, but I'm not sure why. I also think that you don't respect me when you just leave like that.")
4. **SHARE** the feelings you have in response to your thoughts: What emotions are/were you aware of? (e.g. "In response to that I have some fear that if you are upset with me, you will avoid me. I also have some pain and anger- pain

151

because it feels like an old pattern being repeated again, and anger because that felt disrespectful to me."

5. **REQUEST** what need or want that relates to what you have just shared: (e.g. I'd like to request that you not leave so abruptly when we are talking. If you feel like you do need to leave I'd appreciate you at least saying something to let me know what you're doing.")

Note: In Step 3, we highly recommend using phrases such as "What I made up about that in my mind…" or "The meaning I gave to that was…" Using language such as this allows you to take ownership of your reality while leaving plenty of room for your spouse's perspective. It will steer you clear of making outright negative assumptions.

Receiver:

You have one primary goal when your spouse shares his/her reality with you: *Help your spouse feel understood.* You can do that by making eye contact, listening carefully, and not interrupting. You can remind yourself that s/he is *trusting you* by sharing thoughts, feelings and requests. You remind yourself that you are listening to find out where your spouse is at, and more about who s/he is.

As you respect his/her reality, you also connect with your own reality. Use the following steps :

1. **RECOGNIZE** what your spouse just shared. Go as far as you can while remaining authentic. (e.g. "I can understand how you would be feeling those things since that was your experience of what happened.")
2. **SHARE** your reality as it relates to what your spouse has shared. Do you agree or disagree (or both) with what you have just heard? (e.g. "I agree with part of what you've shared, but I disagree with part also. Would you like me to share my perspective?")
3. **RESPOND** to your spouse's request. Look for any part of it you can say "yes" to. Also be clear about what you cannot agree to, or if you would like some time to consider the request. (e.g. "I can certainly agree to try to be more aware of how my leaving the room affects you. I can't promise I'll remember to say something every time, but I can promise you I will try.")

*A word about **Boundary Violations**:* There are certain behaviors that are far outside the spirit of functional intimacy. These behaviors occur when we are unable to contain ourselves and we commit a "boundary violation." These instances need to be confronted and acknowledged. It is as if the "pause" button gets pressed in order to address the boundary violation before moving back into the process of respectfully sharing and receiving. Here are examples:

152

Internal Boundary Violations:
Using sarcastic, demeaning or ridiculing language; eye rolling; yelling or screaming; interrupting; manipulating or controlling; lying

External Physical Boundary Violations:
Touching a person or standing in their personal space without permission; Searching through someone's possessions without permission; eavesdropping on someone's conversations or secretly monitoring email/phone messages

Sexual Boundary Violations:
Engaging a person sexually (physically, verbally or in fantasy) without permission; insisting on having your way sexually when partner says "no;" demanding unsafe sexual practices; exposing others to sexual content/experiences without permission or when inappropriate; sexually shaming someone.

***

You have completed reading this Appendix about Functional Boundaries, but now the real challenge begins: Remembering to use what you have learned and applying it to your day to day life. While it is fine to request that your spouse join you in practicing functional boundaries (and in using the Communication Guidelines), you do not need anyone to do anything in order for YOU to practice functional boundaries. Recalling this truth will help you maintain focus on what you can change. It will help you stay connected to your own power to take care of yourself and to live within your own integrity.

APPENDIX B
Knowing Yourself: Human Sexual Response

"We are all more human than not"
-Harry Stack Sullivan

What is sexually arousing can vary widely from one person to another. However, science has given us some specific ways to understand how we human beings experience the physiological process of sexual arousal. In 1966, Masters and Johnson came forward with their findings from a landmark study of sexual activity in men and women. They concluded that all humans, regardless of the source of arousal or the activity associated with arousal, experienced the same basic bodily responses. They identified four specific stages in this "Sexual Response Cycle:" Excitement, Plateau, Orgasm and Resolution. In the pages that follow, you will read about what is happening in each stage for each gender. It is important to note that what happens in these stages can vary in terms of sensation, duration and fluctuation. It is also the case that moving from one stage to the next can be somewhat less than clearly defined. Furthermore, while there is often a somewhat linear progression through the stages, it is not unusual to have a varied or inconsistent experience of the stages.

> "Sometimes excitement is rapid and leads quickly to orgasm. On other occasions, excitement mounts slowly over a period of hours- while having a romantic, intimate meal, for example- and the rest of the cycle may seem brief in comparison. The plateau stage may not always lead to orgasm as the high levels of arousal that characterize this phase may dissipate and a person may slip back to the excitement phase. If sexual stimulation stops, a person may also drift back into an unaroused state."[30]

Masters and Johnson were careful to emphasize that the "speed, size and strength" of sexual responses is not to be equated with the quality of one's sexual experience or the sexual experience of one's partner.[31] It is remarkable that research done nearly five decades ago is still so widely respected and cited. What follows below is a summary of their model.[13] There have been some recent expansions on their model by other respected sexologists and researchers. These new contributions will be discussed at the end of this section.

---

[13] For further reading, we suggest the outstanding text, *Human Sexuality,* by Masters, Johnson and Kolodny.

154

Human Sexual Response Cycle:

Phase 1: Excitement: In this phase, there is an initial increase in arousal. The following physiological changes occur:

> Women: Vaginal lubrication begins, sometimes not to extent that it is noticeable to the woman; inner two-thirds of vagina expand; the cervix and uterus are pulled upward; outer lips of vagina flatten and move apart; inner lips of vagina enlarge in diameter; clitoris increases in size; nipples may become erect, and breasts may enlarge slightly.

> Men: Penis may become erect, though this can vary widely from completely erect to partially erect to no change at all; the testicles begin to elevate toward the body and increase slightly in size; nipples may become erect.

Phase 2: Plateau: In this phase, the sexual arousal from the excitement phase is continued. Again, there can be considerable variations in duration and subjective experiences of arousal. Arousal may rise gradually through the Plateau stage, or it might build rapidly. In other situations or for other people, arousal may ebb and flow during Plateau. For both genders, there is an increase in muscle tension, heart rates and breathing rates and a small increase in blood pressure. The following physiological changes also occur:

> Women: The tissues in the outer third of the vagina engorge with blood; the inner two-thirds of the vagina expand slightly; uterus becomes elevated; inner labia enlarge, pushing outer labia apart; skin color of inner labia change; clitoris becomes very sensitive as it engorges and retracts under the inner labia; breasts continue to swell and areola enlarges; a spotty "sex flush" may appear on the abdomen or breasts, potentially spreading to other areas of the body (woman is typically unaware)

> Men: Head of penis deepens in color and its diameter near the coronal ridge increases slightly; testicles continue to enlarge and elevate (full elevation indicates orgasm approaching; elevation not as prominent in men over 50 years of age); small amount of fluid may emerge from urethra (it is from the Cowper's glands) and it may contain sperm; warm pressure sensation builds internally around prostate region.

Phase 3: Orgasm: In this phase, the arousal that had been building in the Plateau phase reaches a peak. This is the shortest phase of the sexual response cycle, typically lasting only a matter of seconds. Orgasm is the result of involuntary, rhythmic muscular contractions that produce intense pleasure and a feeling of release of the tension that had been building. Just as in the previous phases, the Orgasm phase also varies in terms of how it is experienced subjectively. Universally, however, heart and breathing rates for both men and women are the highest at any stage in the sexual response cycle during the Orgasm phase. The following physiological changes also occur:

Women: Outer third of vagina and uterus, contract rhythmically and involuntarily (first contractions are intense and rapid, becoming less so as the orgasm continues); foot and facial and hand muscles contract involuntarily.

Men: Vas deferens (tubes in testicles that carry sperm), prostate gland and seminal vesicles begin contracting and force semen into the base of the urethra; rhythmic contractions of the prostate gland along with contractions of the urethra and penis then result in ejaculation (seminal fluid is expelled from the urethra); first contractions are intense and rapid, becoming less so after the first three to four contractions).

Phase 4: Resolution: In the final phase of the sexual response cycle, there are some noticeable differences between genders. Generally speaking, females have the capacity to return to the orgasm phase more efficiently than males, though this varies amongst women. Men are much more predictable in their need for a refractory period before reaching orgasm again, though the length of this period varies among men as well. The physiological changes that occurred during the Excitement and Plateau Stages reverse. Specifically:

Women: The tissues of the labia, clitoris and vagina begin to return to their pre-arousal states: The vagina begins to shorten, the labia return to their normal color, and the clitoris returns to its usual position and size; breasts also decrease in size after orgasm; stimulation of clitoris and vagina may be uncomfortable in the early part of this phase

Men: The penis and testicles return to their pre-arousal states; the testicles descend away from the body, lowering into the scrotum

***

A discussion of sexual response would be incomplete without acknowledging the work of Rosemary Basson, who wrote about a "non-linear" model of sexual response for women[32]. She proposes that women's sexual response varies according to several factors including emotional intimacy, relationship satisfaction and sexual stimuli (e.g spouse initiating something sexual). There are some similarities to the "Circulation Model" you read about in Chapter 5 of this book, though we believe strongly that women *and men* benefit sexually from nurturing their emotional intimacy. This promotes a positive feedback loop between the two types of intimacy which in turn promotes sexual abundance and spiritual intimacy.

Female External Genitalia

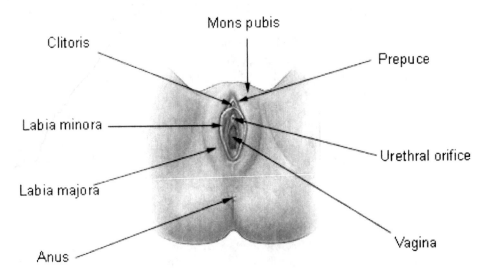

157

Male Genitals

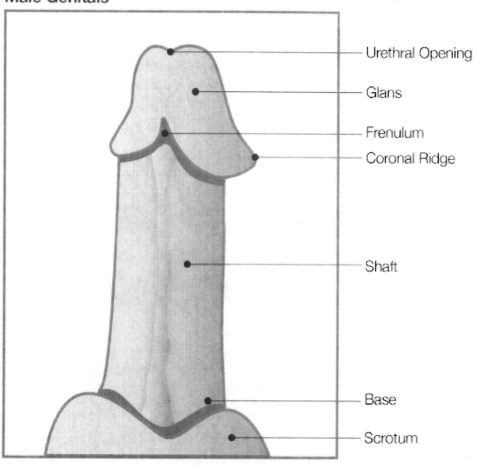

- Urethral Opening
- Glans
- Frenulum
- Coronal Ridge
- Shaft
- Base
- Scrotum

APPENDIX C

Use the chart below to help you schedule each of your Planned Intimate Experiences (PIEs).

Phase I: *Shared Commitment*			
Schedule Date	**PIE**	**Initiator**	**Completed**

Phase II: *Courageous Discovery*			
Schedule Date	**PIE**	**Initiator**	**Completed**

Phase III: *Revelation*			
Schedule Date	**PIE**	**Initiator**	**Completed**

Phase IV: *Enhancement*			
Schedule Date	**PIE**	**Initiator**	**Completed**

Phase V: *Integration*			
Schedule Date	PIE	Initiator	Completed

Bibliography

Adams, Kenneth M., with Alexander P. Morgan. *When He's Married to Mom – How to Help Mother-Enmeshed Men Open Their Hearts to True Love and Commitment.* New York, New York: Simon and Schuster, Inc., 2007.

Black, Claudia. *Deceived: Facing Sexual Betrayal, Lies, and Secrets.* Center City, MN: Hazelden, 2009.

Carnes, Patrick. *Recovery Start Kit.* Carefree, AZ: Gentle Path Press, 2005.

Carnes, Patrick. *The Betrayal Bond: Breaking Free of Exploitive Relationships.* Deerfield Beach, FL: Health Communications, 1997.

Carnes, Patrick. *Out of the Shadows: Understanding Sexual Addiction.* Minneapolis: CompCare Publishers, 1983.

Carnes, Patrick, Laaser, Debra, and Laaser, Mark. *Open Hearts.* Carefree, AZ: Gentle Path Press, 1999.

Carnes, Patrick, with Joseph M. Moriarty. *Sexual Anorexia: Overcoming Sexual Self-Hatred.* Center City, MN: Hazelden, 1997.

Carnes, Stefanie, editor. *Mending a Shattered Heart: A Guide for Partners of Sex Addicts.* Carefree, AZ: Gentle Path Press, 2008.

Corley, M. Deborah, and Jennifer P. Schneider. *Disclosing Secrets: What, to Whom, and How Much to Reveal.* Carefree, AZ: Gentle Path Press, 2002.

Laaser, Debra. *Shattered Vows.* Grand Rapids, MI: Zondervan, 2008.

Laaser, Mark, R. *Healing the Wounds of Sexual Addiction.* Grand Rapids, MI: Zondervan, 1992.

McDaniel, Kelly. *Ready to Heal.* Carefree, AZ: Gentle Path Press, 2008.

Mellody, Pia, with Andrea Wells Miller and J. Keith Miller. *Facing Codependence – What It Is, Where It Comes From, How It Sabotages Our Lives.* New York: HarperCollins, 2003 (reprint).

Mellody, Pia, with Andrea Wells Miller and J. Keith Miller. *Facing Love Addiction: Giving Yourself the Power to Change the Way You Love.* New York: HarperCollins, 1992.

Mellody, Pia, and Lawrence S. Freundlich. *The Intimacy Factor – The Ground Rules for Overcoming the Obstacles to Truth, Respect, and Lasting Love.* New York: HarperCollins, 2003.

Peck, M. Scott. *The Road Less Traveled.* New York: Simon & Schuster, 1992.

Siegel, Daniel and Hartzell, Mary. *Parenting from the Inside Out.* New York: Tarcher/Penguin, 2003.

Weiss, Robert, and Jennifer Schneider. *Untangling the Web: Sex, Porn, and Fantasy Obsession in the Internet Age.* New York, NY: Alyson Books, 2006.

Recommended Reading

Sexual Addiction and Sexual Recovery

Carnes, Patrick. *A Gentle Path through the Twelve Steps: The Classic Guide for All People in the Process of Recovery.* Center City, MN: Hazeldon, 1993.

Carnes, Patrick. *Don't Call It Love: Recovery From Sexual Addiction.* New York: Bantam Books, 1985.

Carnes, Patrick. *Contrary to Love.* Minneapolis, MN: CompCare, 1989.

Carnes, Patrick. *Facing the Shadow: Starting Sexual and Relationship Recovery.* Wickenburg, AZ: Gentle Path, 2001.

Carnes, Patrick, David L. Delmonico, Elizabeth Griffin, with Joseph Moriarity. *In The Shadow of the Net: Breaking Free of Compulsive Online Sexual Behavior.* Center City, MN: Hazelden, 2001.

Carnes, Patrick. *Out of the Shadows.* Minneapolis, MN: CompCare, 1991.

Carnes, Patrick. *Sexual Anorexia.* Center City, MN: Hazelden, 1997.

Corley, M. Deborah, and Jennifer P. Schneider. *Disclosing Secrets: What, to Whom, and How Much to Reveal.* Carefree, AZ: Gentle Path Press, 2002.

Earle, Ralph, and Gregory Crow. *Lonely All the Time.* New York, NY: Pocket, 1989.

Earle, Ralph, and Mark Laaser. *Pornography Trap.* Kansas City, MO: Beacon Hill, 2002.

Ferree, Marnie. *No Stones: Women Redeemed from Sexual Shame.* Revised edition. Downers Grove, Il: InterVarsity Press, 2010.

Laaser, Mark R. *Healing the Wounds of Sexual Addiction.* Grand Rapids, MI: Zondervan, 2004.

Maltz, Wendy and Larry Maltz. *The Porn Trap: The Essential Guide to Overcoming Problems Caused by Pornography.* New York, NY: Harper Collins, 2008.

Schneider, Jennifer. *Back from Betrayal: Recovering from His Affairs.* 3rd edition. Tucson, AZ: Recovery Resources Press, 2005.

Schneider, Jennifer, and Burt Schneider. *Sex, Lies, and Forgiveness: Couples Speak on Healing from Sex Addiction.* 3rd Edition. Tucson, AZ: Recovery Resources Press, 2004.

Weiss, Robert. *Cruise Control: Understanding Sexual Addiction in Gay Men.* Los Angeles, CA: Alyson Books, 2005.

Weiss, Robert, and Jennifer Schneider. *Untangling the Web: Sex, Porn, and Fantasy Obsession in the Internet Age.* New York, NY: Alyson Books, 2006.

Coaddiction/Codependency

Beattie, Melody. *Beyond Codependency.* New York, NY: Harper/Hazelden, 1989.

Beattie, Melody. *Codependent No More.* New York, NY: Harper/Hazelden, 1987.

Black, Claudia. *Deceived: Facing Sexual Betrayal, Lies, and Secrets.* Center City, MN: Hazelden, 2009.

Carnes, Patrick J. *The Betrayal Bond: Breaking Free of Exploitive Relationships.* Deerfield Beach, FL: Health Communications Inc., 1997.

Carnes, Stefanie, editor. *Mending a Shattered Heart: A Guide for Partners of Sex Addicts.* Carefree, AZ: Gentle Path Press, 2008.

McDaniel, Kelly. *Ready to Heal – Women Facing Love, Sex, and Relationship Addiction.* Carefree, AZ: Gentle Path Press, 2008.

Means, Marsha. *Living with Your Husband's Secret Wars.* Grand Rapids, MI: Revell, 1999.

Mellody, Pia and Andrea Wells Miller. *Breaking Free: A Recovery Workbook for Facing Codependence.* San Francisco, CA: Harper, 1989.

Mellody, Pia, with Andrea Wells Miller and J. Keith Miller. *Facing Codependence: What It Is, Where It Comes From, and How It Sabotages Our Lives.* San Francisco, CA: Harper, 2003.

Mellody, Pia with Andrea Wells Miller and J. Keith Miller. *Facing Love Addiction: Giving Yourself the Power to Change the Way You Love.* San Francisco, CA: Harper, 2003.

Mellody, Pia and Lawrence S. Freundlich. *The Intimacy Factor: The Ground Rules for Overcoming the Obstacles to Truth, Respect, and Lasting Love.* San Francisco, CA: Harper, 2003.

Woititz, Janet Geringer, and Garner, Alan. *Lifeskills for Adult Children*. Deerfield Beach, FL: Health Communications, Inc., 1990.

Family-of –Origin

Adams, Kenneth. *Silently Seduced: When Parents Make Their Children Partners – Understanding Covert Incest*. Deerfield Beach, FL: Health Communications, 1991.

Adams, Kenneth. *When He's Married to Mom: How to Help Mother-Enmeshed Men Open Their Hearts to True Love and Commitment*. New York, NY: Simon and Schuster, 2007.

Bassoff, Evelyn S., *Mothering Ourselves – Help and Healing for Adult Daughters*. New York, NY: Penguin Group, 1991.

Black, Claudia. *It Will Never Happen to Me*. New York, NY: Ballantine Books, 1981.

Black, Claudia. *Changing Courses*. Center City, MN. Hazeldon, 1993, 1999.

Love, Patricia, and Jo Robinson. *The Emotional Incest Syndrome: What to Do When a Parent's Love Rules Your Life*. New York: Bantam Books, 1991.

Miller, Alice. *The Drama of the Gifted Child*. New York, NY: Basic Books, Inc., 1981.

Parrott III, Les and Parrott Sr., Les. *The Life You Want Your Kids to Live*. Kansas City, MO: Beacon Hill Press, 2001.

Saltz, Gail. *Becoming Real – Defeating the Stories We Tell Ourselves that Hold Us Back*. New York: Riverhead Books, 2004.

Woititz, Janet Geringer. *Adult Children of Alcholics*. Deerfield Beach, FL: Health Communications, Inc., 1983.

Woititz, Janet Geringer. *Struggle for Intimacy*. Deerfield Beach, FL: Health Communications, Inc., 1990.

Sexual Education and Enrichment

Amen, Daniel G. *Sex on the Brain: 12 Lessons to Enhance Your Love Life*. New York, NY: Three Rivers Press, 2007.

Bader, Michael J. *Arousal: The Secret Logic of Sexual Fantasies.* New York, NY: Thomas Dunn Books, 2002.

Heiman, Julia, and Joseph LoPiccolo. *Becoming Orgasmic: A Sexual and Personal Growth Program for Women.* New York, NY: Simon & Schuster, 1988.

Kaplan, Helen Singer. *How to Overcome Premature Ejaculation.* Florence, KY: Taylor & Francis, 1989.

Love, Patricia, and Jo Robinson. *Hot Monogamy: Essential Steps to More Passionate, Intimate Lovemaking.* New York, NY: Plume, 1995.

McCarthy, Barry, and Michael E. Metz. *Men's Sexual Health: Fitness for Satisfying Sex.* New York, NY: Routledge, 2008.

Metz, Michael E., and Barry W. McCarthy. *Coping with Premature Ejaculation: Overcome PE, Please Your Partner & Have Great Sex.* Oakland, CA: New Harbinger, 2003.

Penner, Clifford and Joyce Penner. *52 Ways to Have Fun, Fantastic Sex: A Guidebook for Married Couples.* Nashville, TN: Thomas Nelson Publishers, 1994.

Penner, Clifford L. and Joyce J. Penner. *Getting Your Sex Life Off to a Great Start: A Guide for Engaged and Newlywed Couples.* Dallas: Word Publishing, 1994.

Penner, Clifford L. and Joyce J. Penner. *Restoring the Pleasure: Complete Step-by-Step Programs to Help Couples Overcome the Most Common Sexual Barriers.* Nashville, TN: W Publishing Group, 1993.

Penner, Clifford and Joyce Penner. *Sex 101: Getting Your Sex Life Off to a Great Start.* Nashville, TN: W Publishing Group, 2004.

Penner, Clifford L. and Penner, Joyce J. *The Gift of Sex: A Guide to Sexual Fulfillment.* Dallas, TX: Word Publishing, 1981.

Penner, Clifford L. and Penner, Joyce J. *The Way to Love Your Wife: Creating Greater Love and Passion in the Bedroom.* Carol Stream, IL: Tyndale House Publishers, 2007.

Schnarch, David. *Passionate Marriage: Love, Sex, and Intimacy in Emotionally Committed Relationships.* New York, NY: Henry Holt and Company, 1997.

Schnarch, David. *Resurrecting Sex.* New York, NY: Harper Collins Publisher, 2002.

Couples Communication and Intimacy

Chapman, Gary. *The Five Love Languages: How to Express Heart-Felt Commitment to Your Mate.* Chicago, IL: Northfield Publishing, 1992.

Fisher, Helen. *Why We Love: The Nature and Chemistry of Romantic Love.* New York, NY: Henry Holt and Company, 2004.

Gottman, John. *Why Marriages Succeed or Fail – and How You Can Make Yours Last.* New York: Simon & Schuster, 1994.

Gottman, John M., and Nan Silver. *The Seven Principles for Making Marriage Work: A Practical Guide from the Country's Foremost Relationship Expert.* New York, NY: Three Rivers Press, 2000.

Hendrix, Harville. *Getting the Love You Want: A Guide for Couples.* New York: Owl Books: 2001 (reprint).

Laaser, Mark and Debra Laaser. *The Seven Desires of Every Heart.* Grand Rapids, MI: Zondervan, 2008.

Lerner, Harriet. *The Dance of Intimacy – A Woman's Guide to Courageous Acts of Change in Key Relationships.* New York: HarperCollins, 1989.

Real, Terrence. *How Can I Get Through to You? Closing the Intimacy Gap Between Men and Women.* New York, NY: Simon & Schuster, 2002.

Real, Terrence. *The New Rules of Marriage: What You Need to Know to Make Love Work.* New York, NY: Ballantine Books, 2008.

Sexual Abuse Recovery

Bass, Ellen and Laura Davis. *Beginning to Heal: A First Book for Men and Women Who Were Sexually Abused as Children.* Revised Edition. New York, NY: Collins, 2003.

Bass, Ellen, and Laura Davis. *The Courage to Heal: A Guide for Women Survivors of Child Sexual Abuse.* 20th Anniversary edition. New York, NY: Harper Collins, 2008.

Lew, Mike. *Victims No Longer: The Classic Guide for Men Recovering froSm Sexual Child Abuse.* 2nd edition. New York, NY: Harper Collins, 2004.

Maltz, Wendy. *The Sexual Healing Journey: A Guide for Survivors of Sexual Abuse.* Revised edition. New York, NY: Harper Collins, 2001.

Acknowledgements

We would like to express our sincere gratitude to the many wonderful people who have supported us in creating this book. First of all, we would like to thank our mentors and friends, Dr. Clifford and Joyce Penner. So much of our Sexual Reintegration Therapy (SRT) program rests solidly upon their substantial body of work in the field of sex therapy. The Penners generously shared their vast clinical knowledge with us when we were newly licensed psychologists who knew very little about what it takes to provide clients with excellent care. The training we received from them has strongly influenced our "therapist instincts." The energy and productivity they modeled has been a wonderful inspiration to us.

Among the most influential people in our personal and professional lives has been Pia Mellody. We have been profoundly affected by her work in the field of emotional trauma resolution. We owe many "functional" experiences to her. We strive to share our understanding of her trauma model with whomever we treat in our practices.

Pia's friend and colleague, Margarita Koutsis, has helped us move toward much healthier versions of ourselves and our marriage than we ever knew were possible. We love her dearly and are grateful for her expert guidance, her investment in us and her abundance of genuine care.

***

One of the most amazing aspects of the process of writing this book has been the outpouring of encouragement we have received from so many of our respected colleagues from coast to coast. Time and again we would hear from people, "My clients need your book – when will it be ready?" This list includes Barbara Levinson, Mavis Humes Baird, Paul & Ginnie Hartman, Ralph Earle, Marcus Earle, Kelly McDaniel, Jennifer Schneider, Alyson Nerenberg, Tom Pecca, Alex Katehakis, Stephanie Carnes, Cara Tripodi, Mari Lee, John & Elaine Leadem, Ken Wells, Steve DeLugach, Mary Linda Sara, Judy Crane, Mark & Debra Laaser, Gino Vaccaro, Nancy Sobel, Marnie Ferree, Sylvia Jason, Ted Roberts, Doug Roseneau, Charlie Riessen, Judy Kelly, Tami Ver Helst, Arlene Story, and John Jamieson.

The production of this book was spearheaded by our incredibly talented and wonderful assistant, Rene Kae Pak. She has worked tirelessly to pull this project together and to allow us to finally cross the finish line. We are lucky to know her and will always remember the focus and dedication she gave to this book.

***

You may have heard the adage, "A little psychology is a dangerous thing." Well, we were introduced to our graduate studies in psychology through a little Masters program in Madison, New Jersey, run by Dr. Herbert Potash and Dr. John Duryee. We will always appreciate their wisdom and guidance during our earliest formative years in this profession. In hindsight, we would amend that old adage to, "Our little psychology program was a wonderful thing!" (And not just because it was where we met!) From there, we were fortunate enough to find Pepperdine University's Doctoral Program in Psychology. This program, led by Dr. Edward Shafranske, Dr. Cary Mitchell, and Dr. Robert de Mayo, gave us the practical experience and theoretical understandings we needed to start forming our own ways of thinking and practicing. It was a stimulating environment in a supportive atmosphere and we will always reflect with gratitude on our time there.

***

We know that any success we have had (or will have) reflects the values and support of our families, including several amazing people who have gone before us. Our parents are responsible for fostering the work ethics within us that allowed us to see this project through. They continue to amaze us with their unwavering support and abundant love.

***

Finally, we would like to thank Patrick Carnes and Rob Weiss in a very special way. We are grateful to know Patrick as a friend and colleague. It is exceptionally rare to find the intellect, passion, vision and humanity that *he* possesses in any one individual. We feel very fortunate that he has shared himself with us as he has. He challenged us to write this book and has been steadfast in his belief that SRT would fill a real treatment need in the recovery community. We thank him for supporting our vision and for his confidence in us. We are tremendously appreciative of his endorsement of this book. We realize that any work we do in this field would not be possible without the light he courageously first shined on a shadowy topic that no one had ever touched before.

We were so fortunate to count on Rob Weiss for guidance and insight throughout our writing process. Rob has helped our writing evolve and has given us some much needed infusions of reassurance along the way. We are truly honored by the Forward he wrote for this book. We hope someday to have a fraction of the positive influence on the recovery community that Rob has had. His efforts to inform public discourse on sexual addiction have been tireless and admirable. We will always be grateful for how high he has set the bar for all of us clinicians and for how generously he has shared his time, energy and passion with us.

***

This book is dedicated to our many brave clients who have entrusted us with their care in the midst of much pain and vulnerability. We hope this book honors your courage.

Additional Acclaim for
The Couple's Guide to Intimacy

"Drs. Bill and Ginger Bercaw have significantly contributed to the field of recovery in sex addiction through their process of Sexual Reintegration Therapy. Their step by step process gives hope to couples who frequently feel hopeless, and leads couples to a deeper spiritual connection as their relationship heals. I highly recommend this book as a very useful tool for couples who are going through the pain of sexual addiction and co-addiction and are ready to work toward healthy intimacy and sexuality in their relationship. I shall be recommending this to our patients at PCS."

> — Ralph Earle, Ph.D., CSAT, Executive Director of Psychological Counseling Services, Ltd., author of *Lonely All the Time*; and *The Pornography Trap*.

"The Bercaws have taken on a topic that is on the minds of many recovering couples that never makes it to the table for discussion in 12 Step meetings and which many addiction professionals shy away from- healthy, sober sexuality. We hope you will let them help you to add a new entry to your gratitude list: *A healthy, intimate sexual relationship!*"

> — John Leadem, MSW, CSAT & Elaine Leadem, MSW CSAT, authors of *One In the Spirit: A Meditation Course for Recovering Couples*

"For those of us who work with trauma and sexual addiction a roar of thanks goes to Drs. Ginger and Bill Bercaw for developing *Sexual Reintegration Therapy* and for sharing it with us. Their powerful book provides a road map for couples not only to heal, but to enrich their intimate relationships in a way that no other material has offered. Through the exercises and assignments we can see how well integrated each piece of work is to the one before and the one after. The material is genuine and simple to understand. I believe that any couple can use this work to deepen and enrich their relationship. Certainly, the couples in pain and anguish that I work with will each receive and use this book for healing. It will be required for all the therapists who practice with me. I am honored to share my excitement with the rest of the therapeutic community and the thousands of couples who will benefit from this book."

> — Judy T. Crane, LMHC, CAP, CSAT, Executive Director of *The Refuge, A Healing Place* (Ocklawaha, FL)

"*The Couple's Guide to Intimacy*, by Drs. Bill and Ginger Bercaw is in itself an integration of several guiding principles from leaders in the field in Sex Addiction, Codependency and Healthy Sexuality. In one book there is both explanation and exercises to help the reader understand and come to terms with the influences that have impacted their sexuality. In a very thoughtful and systematic way, the Bercaws help the reader understand intimacy and build on guided "Personal Intimate Experiences" that teach how to live passionate, healthy erotic lives. This book is a must read for both new and seasoned clinicians, and is a major contribution to the understanding of a very complex issue. Bravo!!"

> — Barbara Levinson Ph.D, RN, LMFT, CSAT, Certified Sex Therapist Diplomate. Founder of *The Center for Healthy Sexuality* (Houston, TX)

"*The Couple's Guide to Intimacy* is a practical, helpful guide to developing both emotional and sexual intimacy. In understandable and straightforward language, the Bercaws present a step-by-step series of lessons that will enable couples to put into action what it takes to achieve the close relationship they have always wanted."

> — Jennifer Schneider, M.D., author of *Sex, Lies & Forgiveness: Couples Speak on Healing from Sex Addiction*

"Drs. Ginger and Bill Bercaw have already established themselves as elite couple's therapists. Their unique approach (using a brilliant technique called *Sexual Reintegration Therapy*) has already helped so many couples recovering from sex addiction. Now that they have found a way to present their healing techniques in book form, many more will know the joy and love that comes from recovery. The Bercaws have created a book that is equally helpful to couples seeking recovery and greater intimacy as well as to therapists who treat them. We enthusiastically recommend their book as required reading for all therapists who treat this population."

> — Ginnie and Paul Hartman, Couples' Therapists and CSAT's, *Pathway to Healing* workshops

"*The Couple's Guide to Intimacy*" will prove to be a significant contribution to the sex addiction recovering community. Ginger and Bill provide the tools for couples to reintegrate a positive, emotionally connected, and respectful sexual experience into their relationship. They enable couples to take what was a hide and seek mentality into a meaningful show and tell functional mindset. Their emphasis on journaling and communication is sure to move couples toward new patterns of sexually relating to one another."

> — Marcus Earle, Ph.D., CSAT, author of *Sex Addiction: Clinical Stories and Case Management*

My wife and I know the devastation of sexual addiction both personally and professionally. Like Ginger and Bill, we have worked with hundreds of couples who struggle to put their sexual lives back together. These couples need guides. The Bercaws are well trained in the disciplines of sex addiction and sex therapy, a perfect combination to offer this guide. Thanks to them for doing it. I heartily recommend it to you."

— Mark Laaser, Ph.D., author of *Healing the Wounds of Sexual Addiction; The Seven Desires of Every Heart; Open Hearts; The Pornography Trap.* Founder of *Faithful and True Ministries* (Eden Prarie, MN)

Endnotes

Chapter One

[1] Patrick Carnes, *Facing the Shadow*, (Carefree, AZ: Gentle Path Press, 2001), 180.

Chapter Two

[2] Patrick Carnes, *CSAT Intensive Training*, April, 2006.

[3] Patrick Carnes, *CSAT Intensive Training*, April, 2006.

[4] Stephanie Carnes, *Mending a Shattered Heart*, (Carefree, AZ: Gentle Path Press), 17.

Chapter Three

[5] Patrick Carnes, *Don't Call it Love: Recovery from Sexual Addiction*, (New York: Bantam Books, 1985).

[6] Patrick Carnes, *Contrary to Love*, (Minneapolis, MN: CompCare, 1989), 127.

[7] Daniel Siegel and Mary Hartzell, *Parenting from the Inside Out* (New York: Tarcher/Penguin, 2003).

Chapter Four

[8] Patrick Carnes, *CSAT Intensive Training*, May, 2006

[9] Pia Mellody, *Post Induction Training*, April/November, *2008*

[10] Pia Mellody, *Post-Induction Training*, April/November, 2008.

[11] Ken Wells, *Recovery Start Kit*, (Carefree, AZ: Gentle Path Press, 2005), 69-105.

[12] Kenneth Adams, (IITAP Conference, personal communication, 2009)

[13] Patrick Carnes, *Sexual Anorexia*, (Center City, NM: Hazelden, 1997), 93.

Chapter Seven

[14] Pia Mellody, *Post Induction Training*, April/November, 2008.

[15] Daniel Siegel. *The Mindful Brain*. (New York: W.W. Norton & Company, Inc.), 31.

[16] Adapted from Dr. Clifford and Joyce Penner, (personal communications, 2001-2009).

Chapter Eight

[17] Adapted from Dr. Clifford and Joyce Penner, (personal communications, 2001-2009).

Chapter Ten

[18] Adapted from Dr. Clifford and Joyce Penner, (personal communications, 2001-2009).

[19] Adapted from Dr. Clifford and Joyce Penner, (personal communications, 2001-2009).

[20] Adapted from Dr. Clifford and Joyce Penner, (personal communications, 2001-2009).

[21] Adapted from Dr. Clifford and Joyce Penner, (personal communications, 2001-2009).

[22] Adapted from Dr. Clifford and Joyce Penner, (personal communications, 2001-2009).

[23] Adapted from Dr. Clifford and Joyce Penner, (personal communications, 2001-2009).

Chapter Eleven

[24] Adapted from Dr. Clifford and Joyce Penner, (personal communications, 2001-2009).

[25] Adapted from Dr. Clifford and Joyce Penner, (personal communications, 2001-2009).

Chapter Twelve

[26] Adapted from Dr. Clifford and Joyce Penner, (personal communications, 2001-2009).

[27] Adapted from Dr. Clifford and Joyce Penner, (personal communications, 2001-2009).

[28] Adapted from Dr. Clifford and Joyce Penner, (personal communications, 2001-2009).

[29] Adapted from Dr. Clifford and Joyce Penner, (personal communications, 2001-2009).

[30] Masters, Johnson & Kolodny, *Human Sexuality*, (New York, NY: Harper Collins College Publishers, Inc., 1995), 74.

[31] Ibid, 75.

[32] Rosemary Basson, Female Sexual Response: The Role of Drugs in the Management of Sexual Dysfunction, *Obstet Gynecol* 2001; 98:350-353

CPSIA information can be obtained at www.ICGtesting.com
Printed in the USA
LVOW09s1728130915

453987LV00017B/653/P